AF267435

CONTAINER GARDENING for BEGINNERS

The Ultimate Starter Guide for Techniques, Tools, and Eco-Friendly Growing

by

Morgan Williams

Bzik Publishing LLC

Seattle, WA

Copyright ©2026 by Morgan Williams

All rights reserved.

No portion of this book may be reproduced, distributed, or transmitted in any form or by any means, including photocopying, recording, or other electronic or mechanical methods, without the prior written permission of the publisher or author, except in the case of brief quotations embodied in critical reviews and certain other noncommercial uses permitted by U.S. copyright law. For permission requests, write to the author through the publisher at the email below.

All included references were accurate at the time of writing and publishing. You are encouraged to conduct your own research and make the best decisions for yourself based on your personal needs.

First printing edition 2026.

All inquiries about this book can be sent to the author via publisher.

Email: BzikPublishing@gmail.com

Bzik Publishing LLC

Seattle, WA

Table of Contents

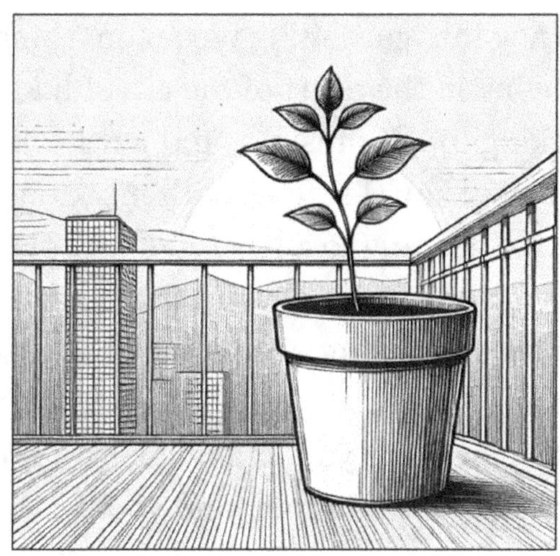

Introduction

Have you ever eagerly planted a balcony full of pots, only to watch them turn into a wilted mess despite your best efforts and an alarming amount of water? If so, you're not alone. Many first-time gardeners, especially those of us with limited space, face similar frustrations. It's easy to think that gardening in small spaces is a lost cause, but I'm here to share some simple garden magic that will change your mind.

"Container Gardening for Beginners" isn't just a book; it's your gateway to transforming tight corners and tiny balconies into lush, productive green spaces. This guide is crafted to demystify the process of container gardening, making it a joyful and rewarding experience, even in the most compact urban environments.

My own journey into gardening began on a small, cluttered balcony in the heart of the city. I had a beautiful view of a parking lot, dumpsters, and a brick retaining wall. Like many of you, I started with more enthusiasm than knowledge, leading to a few too many plant casualties. Over time, through trial and error and countless hours of learning, I discovered the secrets to successful small-space gardening. My mission now is to pass on these insights to you, making sure your gardening story starts off on the right foot, and your plants live to tell the tale!

This book is designed for urban dwellers who crave a slice of nature but might feel restricted by their cramped quarters. Whether you have a tiny patio, a small balcony, or even just a windowsill, this guide will prove that ample space is not a prerequisite for growing beautiful and bountiful plants. The language is simple, the steps are clear, and the tone is light because learning should be as fun as gardening itself.

What sets *"Container Gardening for Beginners"* apart is its focus on practicality and adaptability. You'll find a variety of potting options, essential tips for beginners, innovative irrigation solutions, and a curated list of plants suited for different urban environments. I'll walk you through everything from choosing the right containers and plants to mastering watering techniques that won't leave your balcony flooded or your plants parched. We'll explore how to grow vegetables, herbs, and flowers, and even how to attract pollinators to turn your space into a mini ecosystem.

Approach this book with an open mind and a readiness to experiment. Gardening is not just about growing plants; it's about growing new skills and creating a personal oasis that brings you joy and peace.

Are you ready to transform your limited space into a thriving garden? Let's turn those gardening mishaps into magic. Dig into the pages ahead, and let's start this green journey together!

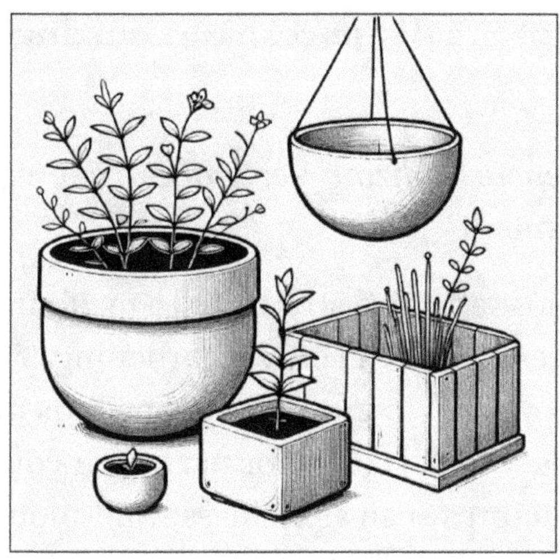

Chapter 1: The Basics of Container Gardening

Gardening in a small urban space often presents a unique set of challenges. However, with the right techniques and knowledge, these obstacles can not only be overcome but can transform your compact living area into a lush, green sanctuary. This chapter is dedicated to unraveling the mysteries of container gardening in confined spaces, particularly focusing on maximizing the limited area of a balcony. As urban dwellers, you may perceive the compactness of your living quarters as a limitation to your gardening aspirations. However, it is possible to cultivate a thriving garden that not only enhances your living space aesthetically but also contributes to your well-being and the environment.

The Magic of Small Spaces: Maximizing Your Balcony

Space Efficiency: Utilizing Vertical Gardening and Hanging Planters

One of the most effective strategies to maximize limited balcony space is through vertical gardening. This approach allows you to grow plants upwards rather than just outwards, which is ideal for narrow or confined areas. Utilizing structures such as trellises, wall-mounted planters, and hanging baskets, you can cultivate a variety of plants without sacrificing valuable floor space. Vertical gardening not only increases your growing area but also adds an element of visual interest and beauty to your urban oasis.

Hanging planters offer another solution for small balconies. These can be suspended from the ceiling or balcony railing, allowing you to utilize overhead space that would otherwise go unused. When selecting plants for hanging planters, consider those with trailing or cascading growth habits, such as ivy, petunias, or ferns, which will create a lush, green canopy overhead. This method not only optimizes space usage but also enhances the aesthetic appeal of your balcony garden.

Microclimate Understanding: Identifying Your Balcony's Unique Environment

Each balcony creates its own microclimate based on factors such as exposure to sun and wind, which affects how plants grow and thrive. To successfully cultivate a balcony garden, it is crucial to assess these environmental conditions. Observe the amount of direct sunlight your balcony receives daily and note any patterns of shade or sun exposure. Additionally, consider the strength and frequency of wind, as balconies on higher floors may experience stronger winds that can stress plants and dry out soil more quickly.

By understanding your balcony's microclimate, you can select plants that are best suited to these conditions, thus increasing your garden's chance of success. For example, balconies that receive full sun are ideal for growing sun-loving herbs and vegetables, while shaded balconies may be better suited to hostas or ferns.

Creative Arrangements: Incorporating Shelves and Tiered Planters

To make the most of your balcony space, consider using shelving units or tiered planters. These structures allow you to arrange plants in a vertically layered way, making efficient use of vertical space. Tiered planters are particularly useful for organizing herbs or smaller plants, which can be grouped aesthetically while still allowing each plant access to sunlight and air circulation.

When arranging plants on shelves or in tiered planters, place taller plants on the lower tiers and shorter or trailing plants on the upper levels to ensure that all plants receive adequate light. Additionally, this arrangement facilitates easy watering and maintenance, as you can access each plant without disturbing others.

Balcony-Specific Challenges: Addressing Wind Protection, Weight Restrictions, and Water Access

Balconies often present specific challenges such as high winds, weight limits, and limited access to water sources. To protect your plants from wind, use heavier containers or secure lighter ones with ties or weights to prevent tipping. Consider wind-resistant plants or use windbreaks such as taller plants, trellises, or decorative screens to shield more sensitive varieties.

Regarding weight restrictions, always check your building's regulations before setting up your garden. Opt for lightweight materials like plastic or resin containers and avoid overloading any single area of your balcony. For water access, if your balcony does not have a nearby faucet, consider setting up a water storage system like a rain barrel or using a watering can to transport water from indoors.

By implementing these strategies, you can transform your balcony into a thriving garden space, proving that even the smallest areas can yield substantial green benefits. Whether you aim to grow a variety of herbs, a selection of ornamental flowers, or a vertical vegetable garden, the principles outlined here will guide you in creating a functional and beautiful green space that enhances your urban home.

Choosing the Right Containers: Material Matters

Selecting the appropriate containers for your urban garden transcends mere functionality; it is pivotal to the success and aesthetics of your plantings. The materials from which these containers are crafted, each come with their distinct advantages and considerations, affecting everything from the health of your plants to the visual appeal of your garden space. Understanding these nuances will guide you in making informed decisions tailored to both your gardening needs and stylistic preferences.

Container materials vary widely, each offering specific benefits and drawbacks. Plastic containers, for instance, are lightweight, cost-effective, and retain moisture well, making them a practical choice for many gardeners operating within small spaces. However, they may not provide the same breathability as more porous materials and can deteriorate under prolonged exposure to sunlight. Conversely, clay pots, renowned for their traditional aesthetics, offer excellent breathability, which helps prevent soil diseases and root rot. Their porous nature allows air and water to move through the walls, promoting healthier root systems. However, clay pots are heavier and more fragile than plastic and tend to dry out more quickly, which can be a challenge for thirsty plants or hotter climates.

Fabric pots are another innovative option that has gained popularity among urban gardeners. These containers are made from breathable fabric, allowing for superior aeration and drainage, leading to robust root growth and preventing issues like root circling in traditional pots. They are also lightweight and can be folded away when not being used, making them ideal for seasonal gardeners with limited storage space. On the downside, fabric pots may require more frequent watering, similar to clay, due to their enhanced breathability. Metal or corrugated tubs, often used for a rustic or industrial look, are durable and can handle a large volume of soil and plants. However, they can conduct heat, potentially overheating the soil on hot days, and may require insulation or placement considerations to mitigate this effect.

The importance of proper drainage in your containers cannot be overstated. Regardless of the material chosen, adequate drainage is crucial to prevent waterlogging, which can lead to root rot and fungal diseases. Ensure that your containers have holes at the bottom or sides to allow excess water to escape. This is essential for maintaining the health of the plant's root systems, which is the foundation of their growth and vitality. For containers that lack pre-made drainage holes, consider drilling your own or using a layer of gravel at the base to promote water flow. However, the latter is less effective at preventing water retention than actual holes.

When selecting the size of the container, it is essential to consider the mature size of the plants you intend to grow. Smaller containers are suitable for herbs and shallow-rooted plants, while larger ones are required for vegetables like tomatoes and shrubs that need more room for their roots to expand. A common mistake is using a container that is too small, leading to cramped roots and stunted growth. Conversely, a container that is too large for a small plant can lead to overly moist soil conditions that could affect plant health. Thus, matching the container size to the plant's needs is critical in setting up your garden for success.

Aesthetically, the choice of container can significantly influence your garden's overall look and feel. Consider the style and color of the containers in relation to the surrounding space. Colorful plastic and glazed ceramic can add a pop of color to a drab balcony, while sleek metal or natural wood finishes complement a more modern aesthetic. The visual coherence of your garden space contributes to its beauty and the pleasure and satisfaction derived from your gardening efforts. Therefore, selecting containers should be thoughtful, harmonizing functional needs with personal style, creating a visually pleasing and thriving garden environment.

The Basics of Soil and Composting in Containers

Soil is the foundation of any garden, container gardens included. The selection of the appropriate soil mix is crucial for the health and growth of your plants. Container gardening requires a special approach to soil because traditional garden soil is too dense, can compact easily, and often doesn't allow adequate root aeration or proper drainage in pots. Instead, a well-balanced, nutrient-rich potting mix that provides good drainage yet retains moisture is needed.

Potting mixes, typically lighter than garden soil, are composed of materials such as peat moss, perlite, and vermiculite. These components help to ensure that the soil is loose enough to allow for good root growth and air circulation yet capable of holding moisture and nutrients. Choosing the right type of potting mix often depends on the types of plants you are growing. For example, succulents and cacti require a mix with more sand or perlite for faster drainage, while moisture-loving plants might benefit from a higher peat moss or coconut coir content. Matching the soil's characteristics with the plant's requirements is imperative to optimize growth and health.

For urban gardeners with limited space, creating your own compost can seem like a challenging task. However, simple composting methods such as bokashi or vermicomposting are well-suited for small spaces and can significantly enrich your potting mix. Bokashi composting, which ferments organic waste in a sealed container, is odorless and quick, making it ideal for apartments. Vermicomposting, which uses worms to break down organic waste, can be done in small bins, providing excellent nutrients for container plants. Incorporating homemade compost into your potting mix recycles kitchen waste and introduces beneficial microorganisms that help plant roots absorb nutrients more effectively.

Maintaining soil fertility in containers over time requires regular attention. Over time, potting soil can become depleted of nutrients as plants absorb them, and the soil structure can degrade, impacting aeration and water retention. To counteract this, it is essential to refresh the soil annually by either replacing a portion of the old soil with new, nutrient-rich mix or by top-dressing with fresh compost. Regular fertilization is also crucial, as container plants do not have the natural sources of nutrients that ground-planted gardens do. Use a balanced, slow-release fertilizer that provides a steady supply of essential nutrients over time. Be mindful of the specific needs of your plants, as over-fertilization can lead to root burn and under-fertilization can cause stunted growth and poor flowering or fruiting.

The health of a plant is fundamentally linked to the health of its roots, which in turn is significantly influenced by the choice of soil. Good potting mix provides a balance of drainage and water-holding capacity, preventing both waterlogged and dried-out conditions, which can stress plants and lead to disease. The structure of the soil also impacts root health by ensuring enough space for roots to grow, breathe, and absorb nutrients efficiently. Compacted or unsuitable soil can choke roots, making plants weak and susceptible to pests and diseases. Therefore, selecting the right soil and maintaining its condition is not just about fostering growth above the ground but ensuring a healthy root system below it.

In container gardening, every choice, from the pot to the plant, hinges significantly on the soil. With the constraints of limited space, ensuring that your soil is meticulously chosen and maintained can make the difference between a struggling garden and a flourishing one. The effort you put into selecting the right soil mix, creating and using compost effectively, and maintaining soil health will directly reflect in the vibrancy and productivity of your urban garden. Understanding and managing soil health is not merely a fundamental aspect of gardening, it is a critical determinant of your garden's success.

Understanding Light: What Your Plants Need

Light is integral to plant life and governs photosynthesis, the process by which plants convert light into energy. Thus, understanding and managing light exposure is crucial for the health and productivity of your garden. For urban gardeners, particularly those dealing with the spatial constraints of balconies or limited outdoor areas, this involves a nuanced approach to how light interacts with their gardening space.

Know Your Zone: Utilizing Hardiness Zone Information

The concept of hardiness zones, developed by the United States Department of Agriculture (USDA), is a standard by which gardeners can determine which plants are most likely to thrive at a location. These zones are defined by the average annual minimum winter temperature, divided into 10-degree F zones. Knowing your hardiness zone is the first step for urban gardeners to select plants that will succeed in your local climate conditions. This information can be particularly invaluable when you are choosing perennials or any plant you hope to cultivate year-round, as these plants must be able to withstand the winter temperatures of your area.

You can easily refer to the USDA's online zone map (https://planthardiness.ars.usda.gov) to find your hardiness zone, where you input your ZIP code to receive your specific zone. Once this is known, you can filter your plant choices, ensuring compatibility with your climate. For instance, if you reside in zone 6, selecting plants rated for zones 3-6 ensures they can survive the winter temperatures typical of your area. This preliminary step optimizes your garden's potential and prevents the disappointment of losing plants to unsuitable climatic conditions.

Light Requirements: Decoding Sunlight Needs for Container Plants

Different plants require varying amounts of light, categorized generally into full sun, partial sun or partial shade, and full shade. Full sun plants thrive with at least six to eight hours of direct sunlight daily, making them ideal for balconies facing south or west. Examples include most vegetables and flowering plants, which need ample light to produce bountiful yields and vibrant blooms. Partial sun or partial shade plants require about three to six hours of sunlight each day and can tolerate some direct sun exposure, especially if it is not during the hottest part of the day. Such conditions are typical for east-facing balconies, where morning light is abundant but not overly harsh. Full shade plants, thriving with less than three hours of direct sunlight daily, are perfect for north-facing balconies or areas shadowed by other buildings, where light is minimal.

Understanding the light requirements of your chosen plants is essential, as improper light exposure can lead to poor growth, lack of flowers or fruit, and increased susceptibility to diseases. When planning your garden, consider the light needs of each plant, aiming to match these needs with the areas of your balcony that meet these conditions.

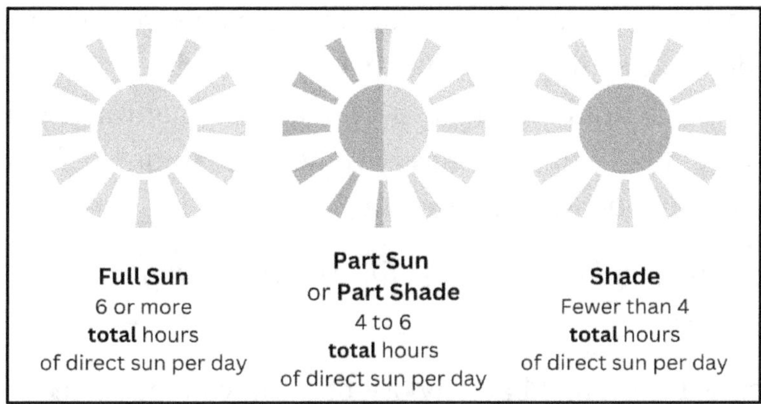

Plant shade requirements

Balcony Orientation: Impact of Direction on Sunlight Exposure

The orientation of your balcony significantly affects the amount of sunlight your garden receives, which in turn influences what types of plants you can successfully grow. South and west facing balconies generally receive the most sunlight, often getting several hours of direct sunlight. This makes them suitable for plants that require full sun. East-facing balconies receive morning sunlight, which is less intense, making them ideal for plants that need partial sun. North-facing balconies, which receive the least light, are well-suited to shade-tolerant plants. West-facing balconies, receiving afternoon sun, can host plants that thrive in either full sun or partial shade, but the intense afternoon heat might be too harsh for some plants, necessitating some form of light diffusion or shading to mitigate the intense exposure.

For urban gardeners, assessing the orientation of your garden space and matching it with appropriate plant choices is a fundamental aspect of garden planning. This ensures that each plant receives the right amount of light, maximizing health and growth.

Adjusting Light: Strategies for Managing Light Exposure

Even with optimal balcony orientation, you may need to adjust light exposure to meet specific plant needs. One effective method is the strategic placement of plants. Taller plants can be placed to shield shorter, more light-sensitive plants from excessive sunlight, naturally creating areas of partial shade. Additionally, reflective surfaces like mirrors or light-colored walls can increase light availability for plants situated in less illuminated areas.

Artificial lighting can provide a supplementary solution for balconies that struggle with low light levels. Grow lights, specifically designed to support plant growth, can help compensate for insufficient natural light, ensuring your plants receive the necessary light spectrum for photosynthesis. These lights are particularly useful during winter months or for balconies with suboptimal light conditions.

Seasonal Changes: Adapting to Varying Light Conditions

Light conditions are not static and change with the seasons. The angle of the sun shifts throughout the year, affecting how much sunlight your balcony receives. When the sun is high in summer, balconies might experience more direct sunlight, while in winter, lower sun angles might reduce light exposure. Recognizing these patterns allows you to anticipate changes and adjust your garden accordingly.

Seasonal adjustments include relocating plants to optimize their light exposure or altering your use of artificial lights. Tracking how sunlight patterns change across seasons on your balcony can help you plan these adjustments effectively, ensuring that your plants consistently receive the right amount of light. This proactive approach to managing light exposure supports the ongoing health of your plants and enhances your overall gardening success, allowing you to enjoy a vibrant and productive garden year-round.

Watering Wisdom: Keeping Your Garden Hydrated

Watering your garden effectively is not merely about providing your plants with water; it is about understanding the unique hydration needs of each plant, recognizing the signs of water stress, and employing techniques that optimize water usage without leading to overwatering or underwatering. This knowledge is crucial, especially in a container gardening setting where the margin for error is often narrower due to the limited soil volume.

Watering Wisely

To water wisely begins with recognizing the signs of water distress in plants. Underwatering typically manifests as drooping leaves, dry and brittle leaf edges, and slow, stunted growth. In severe cases, the lower leaves may turn yellow and drop off, and the soil will feel dry. Conversely, overwatering can lead to the plant's general wilting or sogginess, despite the soil being wet. Leaves may turn darker than normal, often becoming soft and limp. Root rot, indicated by a foul smell coming from the soil, is a common consequence of excessive watering and poor drainage.

Effective watering goes beyond just surface watering. It involves watering deeply and thoroughly, ensuring the water reaches the entire root system. This method encourages deeper root growth, which helps plants access nutrients and moisture even from the lower layers of the container. For most plants, allowing the top inch of soil to dry out before watering again helps prevent over-watering. This technique ensures that the plant's roots have adequate moisture without waterlogging the soil. During hot or windy weather, plants in containers may need more frequent watering, sometimes as often as once a day, because of the increased evaporation rates.

Watering Techniques

Several techniques can help prevent overwatering and underwatering, thereby promoting healthier plant growth. One effective method is using self-watering containers, which have a reservoir at the bottom that allows plants to absorb moisture as needed. This system not only conserves water but also helps maintain consistent moisture levels, which is particularly beneficial for moisture-loving plants and reduces the risk of human error in watering schedules.

Another technique is the use of watering globes or drip irrigation systems, which provide a slow and steady supply of water directly to the roots. This method reduces water wastage and surface evaporation and is ideal for gardeners who cannot water their plants daily. For those who prefer manual watering, using a watering can with a long spout helps direct the water to the base of the plant, minimizing moisture loss and ensuring that water reaches the root zone where it is most needed.

Moisture Monitoring

Monitoring soil moisture is key to understanding when your plants need water. Tools such as soil moisture meters can be invaluable. These devices, which measure the soil's moisture level, provide a more accurate indication than simply touching the soil. They can be especially helpful for beginner gardeners who may not yet be able to judge soil moisture simply by feel. Alternatively, a simple method is using a wooden stick or even a finger to check the moisture level; if the stick or finger comes out clean without any soil sticking, it is likely time to water.

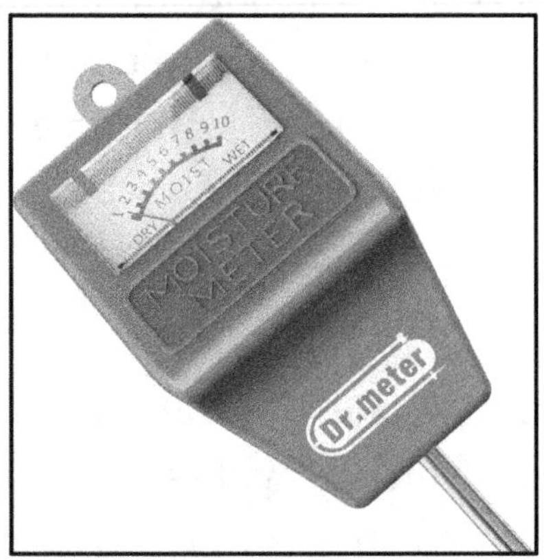

Moisture meter

Watering Schedule

Creating a watering schedule that considers the plants' needs and environmental factors is vital. While many gardening guides suggest watering schedules, such as watering twice a week, the truth is that the ideal frequency depends on several factors, including the type of plant, the stage of growth, the weather, and the quality of the soil. For example, young seedlings may need frequent, lighter watering to keep the soil consistently moist, whereas established plants may prefer less frequent, but deeper watering. Keeping a garden journal where you record watering times, weather conditions, and plant health can help you adjust your watering strategy to meet your garden's specific needs better.

Drought-Resistant Plants

Choosing drought-resistant plants can be a practical solution for gardeners who may not be able to maintain a consistent watering schedule. Species such as sedum, lavender, and succulents are well-suited to conditions where water is scarce. These plants have adapted to survive in dry environments by storing moisture in their leaves or roots and developing deep root systems to access water deeper in the soil. Incorporating these plants into your garden reduces the need for frequent watering and adds variety and interest to your plant collection.

Understanding and implementing effective watering practices is crucial in container gardening, where each choice can significantly impact plant health. You can ensure that your garden remains vibrant and healthy by recognizing the signs of improper watering, employing efficient watering techniques, monitoring soil moisture accurately, and adjusting watering schedules based on real-time conditions. Additionally, choosing plants that are well-suited to your watering capabilities can minimize maintenance while maximizing the beauty and productivity of your garden space.

The Art of Fertilizing: Nutrients for Your Container Garden

Understanding and managing the nutritional needs of your container garden is paramount to fostering robust plant growth and bountiful yields. Plants in containers rely solely on the nutrients provided in their confined soil, which can be depleted rapidly compared to in-ground gardens. This makes it crucial to grasp the types of nutrients your plants require and the signs of deficiencies that may arise when these needs are not adequately met.

Plants require a variety of nutrients, categorized into macronutrients and micronutrients. Macronutrients, including nitrogen (N), phosphorus (P), and potassium (K), are needed in larger quantities. Nitrogen is vital for leaf and stem growth and gives leaves their green color. A deficiency might manifest as yellowing leaves and stunted growth. Phosphorus is crucial for energy transfer and photosynthesis within the plant, promoting root and flower development; a lack of phosphorus can result in stunted growth and darkened or purplish leaves. Potassium helps in the overall functions of the plant, such as protein synthesis and water absorption, with deficiencies typically showing as brown scorching and curling at the leaf edges. Although required in smaller amounts, micronutrients, including elements like iron, manganese, and zinc are equally vital, affecting the plant's health and ability to withstand diseases and pests.

When purchasing fertilizer, both organic and synthetic, the N-P-K numbers, such as 10-10-10 or 20-5-10, tell you the percentage by weight of each nutrient. For example, in a 100-pound bag of 10-10-10 fertilizer, there would be 10 pounds each of nitrogen, phosphorus, and potassium. The remaining weight is usually composed of other nutrients or inert materials. Choosing the right N-P-K ratio depends on your specific gardening needs, the type of plants you are growing, and the existing soil conditions.

The choice between organic and synthetic fertilizers can significantly impact the health of your garden and the environment. Organic fertilizers, derived from natural sources such as compost, manure, or bone meal, release nutrients slowly as they break down in the soil. This provides a steady nutrient supply, enhances the soil structure, and encourages beneficial microbial activity. However, the nutrient ratios in organic fertilizers can vary, making precise nutrient management challenging. On the other hand, synthetic fertilizers are manufactured with specific nutrient ratios and are readily available to plants almost immediately upon application. While they offer the advantage of precise control over nutrient delivery, their rapid release can sometimes lead to nutrient runoff, which may harm the environment. Additionally, overuse can lead to salt buildup in the soil, potentially damaging plant roots.

Proper application of fertilizer is crucial to avoid damaging your plants. Over-fertilizing can be just as detrimental as under-fertilizing, potentially leading to nutrient burn or even plant death. When applying fertilizer, ensure that it is evenly distributed across the soil and never concentrated at the base of the plant, as this can burn the roots. For granular fertilizers, lightly mix them into the top layer of soil or follow the specific instructions provided on the package. Liquid fertilizers, often preferred for their ease of use and quick action, should be diluted as directed and applied to the soil, not the foliage, to prevent leaf burn.

Creating a fertilizing schedule tailored to the growth stages of your plants and the seasonal changes in their growth cycle is essential for optimal plant health. In general, most plants benefit from increased fertilization during their peak growing periods in the spring and summer, when they are actively growing and using nutrients rapidly. During these times, a balanced fertilizer, typically one with equal proportions of nitrogen, phosphorus, and potassium, can promote healthy growth and flowering. As the growing season winds down in the fall, reduce the frequency of fertilization to prepare the plants for dormancy. Winter fertilization is usually not necessary unless you are growing winter crops or indoor plants that continue to grow actively during the colder months.

In container gardening, the balance of nutrients is vital for plant health and productivity. By understanding the specific nutrient needs of your plants, choosing the right type of fertilizer, applying it correctly, and adhering to a thoughtful fertilizing schedule, you can ensure that your plants have the necessary resources to thrive. This approach not only maximizes the health and yield of your garden but also contributes to creating a sustainable and environmentally friendly gardening practice.

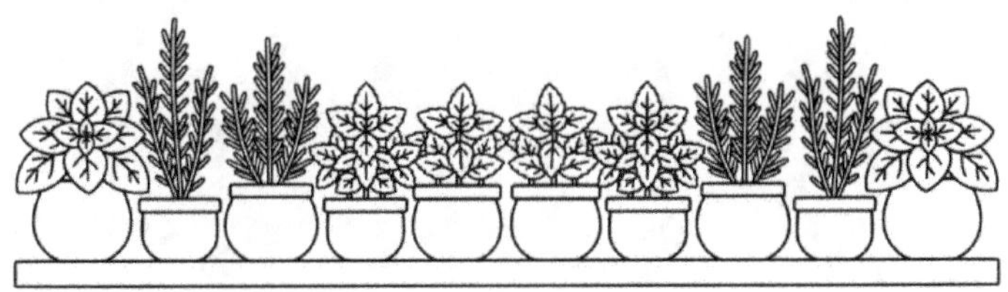

Key Chapter 1 Takeaways:

- Use vertical strategies such as trellises, shelves, tiered planters, and hanging containers to increase growing space without crowding the floor.

- Observe your balcony's microclimate, including sun exposure, wind, and seasonal changes, before selecting plants.

- Choose containers based on material, size, weight limits, and drainage to support healthy root systems.

- Use a quality potting mix designed for containers and refresh nutrients regularly with compost or fertilizer.

- Match plants to available light and watering conditions rather than trying to force unsuitable plants to adapt.

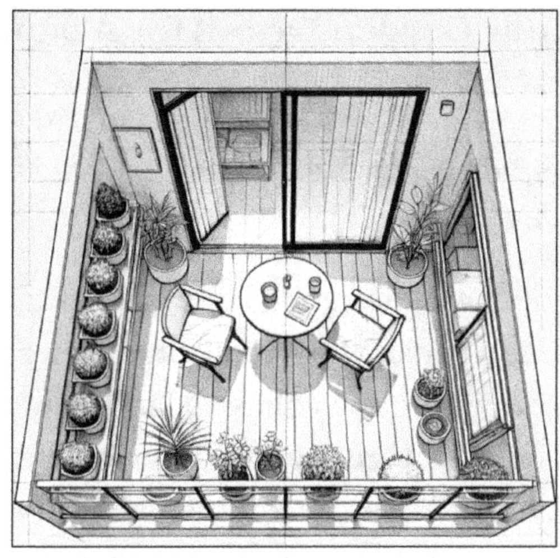

Chapter 2: Designing Your Container Garden

Embarking on creating a container garden transforms your urban space into a sanctuary where aesthetics meet productivity. This chapter guides you through the foundational principles of garden layout design that ensure visual appeal and promote healthy plant growth. The design of your garden should reflect your personal style while maintaining functionality for plant health and growth. This delicate balance requires careful planning and a thoughtful approach.

Planning Your Garden Layout for Aesthetics and Growth

Design Principles: Crafting a Visually Cohesive Container Garden

The essence of a well-designed container garden lies in its ability to create a sense of harmony and order, drawing the observer's eye across a cohesive landscape. This visual harmony is achieved through the thoughtful application of basic design principles, including balance, contrast, repetition, and scale. Balance ensures that the garden feels stable and proportioned, which can be achieved symmetrically or asymmetrically, depending on your personal preference. Contrast can be introduced through variations in color, texture, or form, providing visual interest and focal points. Repetition strengthens a design by tying disparate elements together with consistent patterns or themes, be it through repeating similar plant types or container styles. Lastly, understanding scale involves selecting plants and containers that are proportional to the space available, ensuring that the garden components do not overwhelm the space or seem too insignificant.

Space Utilization: Maximizing Aesthetics and Growth in Limited Areas

In urban environments where space is at a premium, every inch counts. Effective space utilization involves more than just maximizing the number of plants in an area; it requires strategic planning to ensure each plant receives enough light, air, and nutrients to thrive. This might mean choosing a variety of containers that can be efficiently arranged to take advantage of vertical space, such as using hanging baskets or tiered plant stands. Additionally, consider the growth habits of the plants chosen. Some plants, like climbing vines, can be trained up trellises, thus using vertical space that would otherwise go unused. Others, such as sprawling bush-type plants, may require more horizontal space and should be placed where they can spread without crowding their neighbors.

Visual Height: Creating Dynamic Impact

Incorporating elements of varying heights can dramatically enhance the visual appeal of your garden, creating layers that draw the eye upward and maximize the use of space. This can be achieved through a mix of tall plants, medium-sized plants, and ground covers or the strategic placement of containers themselves on stands or stacked arrangements. However, it's crucial to consider the visual background, or the area against which your garden is set. Tall elements should not block natural light sources or overpower the scene but rather complement the existing backdrop. When planning the layout, visualize the garden from different angles to ensure that taller elements enhance the space without dominating it.

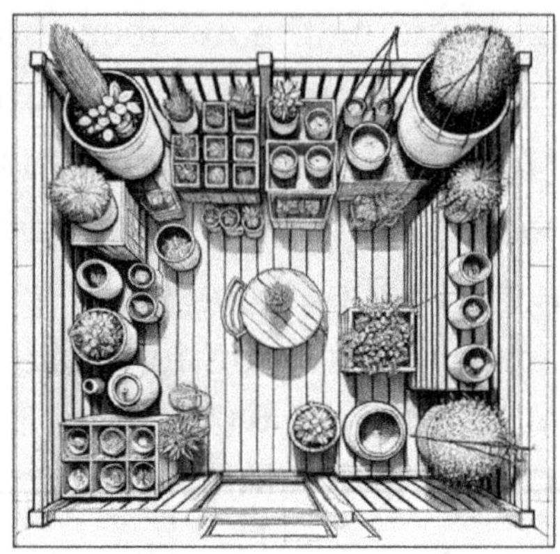

Growth Patterns: Anticipating Future Growth

A common oversight in garden planning is underestimating the growth potential of plants. During the design phase, it's essential to consider not only the current size of the plants but also their mature sizes. This foresight prevents future issues such as overcrowding, which can inhibit growth and lead to health problems like poor air circulation and reduced light exposure. Each plant's growth pattern, whether upright, sprawling, or compact, should inform its placement in the garden layout. Plants that are likely to spread wide might be better positioned at the edges of your space or in larger containers, while upright, narrow plants can be placed where they won't obstruct views or interfere with other plants.

Color Schemes and Plant Selection

Color Coordination: Crafting a Harmonious Palette

The thoughtful selection of colors in your container garden not only enhances the visual appeal of your space but can also influence the mood and atmosphere of your urban oasis. When choosing plant colors, consider the existing colors of your home's exterior and furnishings to create a cohesive look. A harmonious color palette can be achieved by selecting plants whose blooms or foliage complement or subtly contrast with these background hues. For instance, if your outdoor furniture features cool blue tones, planting containers with flowers in varying shades of violets and blues can enhance this serene color scheme. Conversely, for a vibrant, energizing effect, opt for plants with blooms in warm tones like reds, yellows, and oranges.

It is also beneficial to consider the psychological impacts of color. Cooler colors such as blue, green, and purple tend to create a calming atmosphere, ideal for relaxation spaces. Warmer colors, on the other hand, evoke feelings of warmth and excitement, which might be preferable in entertainment areas. In addition to aesthetic compatibility, consider the lighting of your garden space. Some colors show up brilliantly in bright sunlight, while others are more visible in shade or during dusk hours, offering opportunities to play with light and shadow through your color choices.

Seasonal Colors: Ensuring Year-Round Vibrancy

Maintaining visual interest throughout the year requires strategically choosing plants that bloom or change color in different seasons. For continuous color, integrate a mix of annuals, which will bloom for one season and then need to be replanted, and perennials, which return year after year. Spring might shine with the soft pastels of tulips and cherry blossoms, while summer could bring the bold reds and yellows of marigolds and sunflowers. Consider adding chrysanthemums or ornamental kale in autumn, which offer deep russets and purples, reflecting the changing foliage. For winter interest, plants like holly, with its bright red berries or evergreen shrubs, can add color and texture even in colder months.

This approach not only ensures that your garden remains attractive all year round but also helps you plan gardening activities throughout the year, keeping you engaged with your space. It's crucial to research the bloom times and duration of color for each plant you consider to ensure that your garden transitions smoothly from one season to the next without losing its visual appeal.

Foliage vs. Flowers: Balancing Beauty

While blooms are often the stars of the show, foliage should not be overlooked for its ability to add depth and continuity to your garden's color scheme. Plants with interesting or variegated foliage can provide a backdrop that highlights the seasonal blooms or stand on their own for year-round color. For example, the silver tones of dusty miller or the deep purples of heuchera can provide a stunning contrast to green leaves, bringing a sophisticated palette to your space.

Moreover, some plants offer spectacular flowers and striking foliage, giving you the best of both worlds. Balancing flowering plants with those known for their colorful foliage ensures that your garden remains vibrant even when blooms are absent. This strategy is particularly useful in extending visual interest beyond the blooming season, ensuring your garden remains visually appealing throughout the year.

Theme Gardens: Creating Focused Visual Stories

Theme gardens can be a delightful way to express creativity and personalize your space. Whether you choose an all-edible garden that combines various herbs and vegetables in aesthetically pleasing arrangements, a monochromatic theme using varying shades of a single color, or a pollinator-friendly garden designed to attract bees and butterflies, each theme can offer a unique visual and sensory experience. When planning a theme garden, consistency is key. Choose plants that not only support the theme but also thrive in the conditions of your garden.

An all-edible garden, for instance, combines functionality with aesthetic appeal, providing fresh produce while also adding color and variety to your space. Monochromatic gardens can create a striking visual impact using plants of different textures and forms but similar colors. Meanwhile, pollinator gardens add beauty, interest, and support local wildlife, contributing to biodiversity. Each theme offers a way to unify your gardening efforts under a single visual and conceptual banner, making your gardening practice both focused and satisfying.

By carefully selecting color schemes, considering seasonal changes, balancing the use of foliage and flowers, and potentially adopting a thematic focus, you can transform your container garden into a dynamic part of your urban home. Each decision not only enhances the beauty of your space but also supports the growth and health of the plants, creating a sustainable and engaging garden environment.

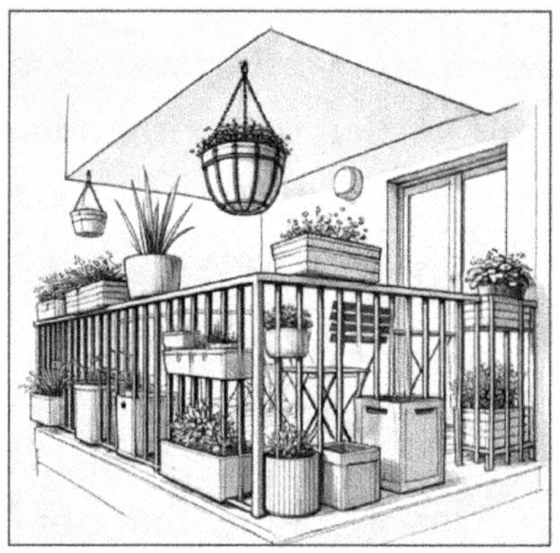

Incorporating Vertical Gardening into Your Space

Vertical gardening, an innovative approach to horticulture, is particularly suited to urban environments where horizontal space may be limited. This method extends the gardening plane vertically, using walls, trellises, and other structures. Thus, it provides an excellent solution for those looking to maximize their green areas without sacrificing valuable floor space. Understanding the types of structures available and the specific plants that thrive in vertical conditions is crucial for anyone looking to explore this dynamic gardening style.

Vertical Structures: Exploring Options for Vertical Gardening

Several structures can facilitate vertical gardening, each offering unique advantages depending on your specific needs and space constraints. Trellises are among the most popular choices; these lattice-like frameworks support climbing plants and can be made from wood, metal, or plastic. They can be freestanding or attached to walls, providing flexibility in placement and use. Another effective vertical structure is the wall planter, which consists of containers affixed directly to a wall. These can range from simple pot holders to sophisticated modular systems that allow for extensive customization. Wall planters are particularly effective for creating living walls that can transform a bare exterior into a lush, verdant surface.

Other vertical gardening options include tiered hanging baskets, which are suspended from balconies or ceilings,

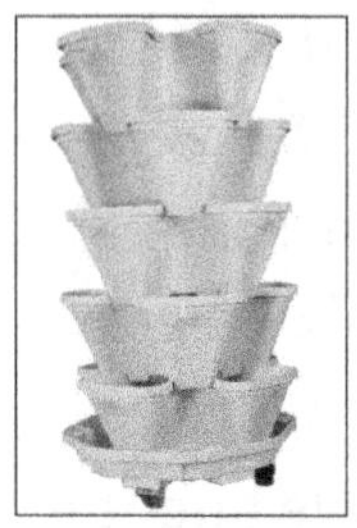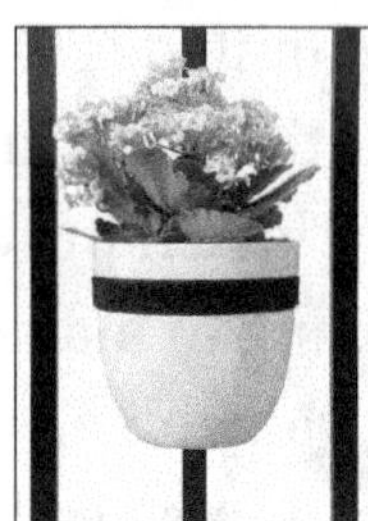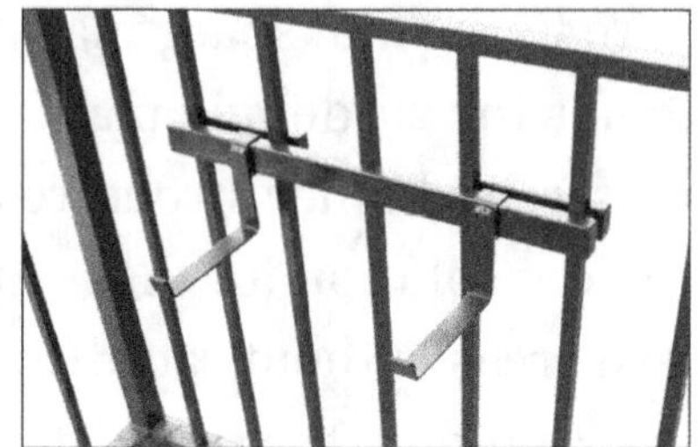

Examples of vertical garden and balcony mounted options

and vertical stacking planters, which allow plants to be arranged in a cascading vertical tower. Each of these options utilizes vertical space efficiently, enabling you to grow a variety of plants in a compact area. When selecting a vertical structure, consider factors such as weight capacity, material durability, and ease of installation, as well as how the structure will integrate with the overall aesthetic of your space.

Plant Choices: Selecting Suitable Plants for Vertical Gardening

Not all plants are suited to vertical growth; selecting the correct species is critical to a thriving vertical garden. Climbing plants such as ivy, clematis, and jasmine are natural choices for trellises and arches, as they have tendrils that cling to structures, allowing them to grow upwards effortlessly. These plants can cover large areas relatively quickly, providing lush, dense foliage that can act as a privacy screen while adding beauty to your urban oasis.

For wall planters, consider plants with a more compact growth habit, such as ferns, begonias, and certain herbs like basil and thyme. These plants do not require extensive root space, making them ideal for the confined soil volumes of wall containers. Succulents are another excellent option for vertical wall gardens; their low water needs and shallow root systems make them well-suited to the limited soil depth in typical wall planters. Additionally, their variety of forms and colors can create visually striking patterns, enhancing the decorative appeal of your garden.

DIY Solutions: Creating Cost-Effective Vertical Gardens

Numerous DIY solutions can be employed for those on a budget to create effective vertical gardening structures. Pallet gardens are a popular and eco-friendly option, utilizing reclaimed wooden pallets as a frame for growing plants. By adding landscape fabric to the back and sides of the pallet and filling it with soil, you can plant directly into the slats, creating a vertical display of herbs, flowers, or greens. Ensure that the pallet you are using has not been chemically treated. Some pallets are treated with chemicals to prevent rot and insect damage, which are toxic to human consumption. Another simple DIY approach is using upcycled containers such as old bottles, cans, or even shoes, which can be attached to a fence or wall to serve as unique plant holders. Ensure that the edges of the bottles or cans are rounded or dull to prevent personal harm.

These DIY projects save money and allow you to customize your garden to your specific tastes and needs. They can be particularly rewarding, giving you a sense of accomplishment and a deep connection to your gardening space.

Maintenance Tips: Caring for Your Vertical Garden

Maintaining a vertical garden involves considerations similar to those of traditional gardening but adapted to the vertical setup. Watering, for example, needs careful attention, as gravity causes water to drain downward more quickly in vertical planters, potentially leading to uneven moisture distribution. Drip irrigation systems can be particularly useful in these setups, delivering water directly to the roots of each plant and ensuring that all plants receive adequate hydration.

Pruning is another important maintenance aspect, especially for fast-growing climbers that can become unruly if left unchecked. Regular pruning not only keeps your plants within bounds but also encourages healthier, thicker growth. It is also important to monitor for pests and diseases, as the close proximity of plants in vertical gardens can sometimes facilitate the spread of issues. Regular inspections and prompt treatment of any problems will help keep your vertical garden healthy and vibrant.

Employing these strategies can ensure that your vertical garden remains not only a stunning focal point of your living space but also a flourishing environment for a variety of plants. Through careful planning, appropriate plant selection, innovative DIY projects, and diligent maintenance, your vertical garden will transform any small urban space into a lush, verdant retreat.

Balcony Beautification with Edible Plants

Edible and Aesthetic: Cultivating Beauty and Utility in Urban Gardens

In the quest to create a garden that is both functional and visually appealing, incorporating edible plants that also possess ornamental qualities can offer a dual-purpose solution, especially in urban settings where space is at a premium. Edible plants are productive, providing fresh produce right at your doorstep, and many varieties also bring striking visual interest to your garden. For instance, Swiss chard, with its brightly colored red, pink, or yellow stems, adds a vibrant splash of color, while purple varieties of basil contribute lush, dark foliage that can contrast beautifully against lighter greens. Similarly, peppers come in various colors and shapes, from the glossy sheen of bell peppers to the fiery allure of chili peppers, each adding a unique aesthetic element to your balcony garden.

Integrating such plants requires a thoughtful approach to maximize their visual attributes without compromising their edible yield. Positioning is key; place plants where they can receive the appropriate amount of sunlight needed to thrive while also considering how they appear to one another. A palette of edible plants can be coordinated like a flower garden, using color and form to create a cohesive look. For example, the silvery foliage of sage can complement the deep purples of opal basil, while the bright greens of lettuce create a fresh, lively backdrop. This careful arrangement enhances the balcony's aesthetic and encourages regular maintenance and harvesting, as the appealing setup invites interaction and enjoyment.

Herb Gardens: Enhancing Culinary and Visual Delights

Herb gardens are particularly suited to balcony settings due to herb plants' generally compact nature and their diverse textures, colors, and aromas. Cultivating a selection of herbs offers a practical and sensory-rich garden component. From the soft, fine leaves of dill to the robust, glossy foliage of bay laurel, herbs can be selected to create a tapestry of textures and hues. Moreover, herbs like lavender and rosemary produce flowers that attract pollinators, adding another layer of visual and ecological value to your garden.

The utility of herbs extends beyond their beauty, as they provide fresh flavors for cooking and can be harvested as needed, ensuring maximum freshness and reducing food waste. Consider their growth requirements and harvest cycles to make the most of these culinary assets. Many herbs, including basil and cilantro, prefer full sun, while others, like parsley and mint, can tolerate partial shade, which allows for strategic placement within the balcony's microclimate. Grouping herbs with similar watering needs together simplifies maintenance and can help prevent overwatering or underwatering, enhancing plant health and productivity.

Fruit-Bearing Plants: Compact Varieties for Container Cultivation

Growing fruit on a balcony may seem ambitious, but many compact and dwarf varieties of fruit trees and shrubs are well-suited to container gardening. Dwarf citrus trees, such as lemons and limes, provide fragrant flowers and edible fruit and have an attractive form that can serve as a focal point in your garden design. Similarly, strawberry plants offer visual appeal and sweet rewards with bright red berries and delicate flowers. These plants can be grown in hanging baskets or tiered planters, utilizing vertical space effectively and adding depth to your garden's layout.

When selecting fruit-bearing plants for your balcony, consider their pollination needs and fruiting seasons. Some fruits, like self-pollinating blueberries, are easier to grow in isolation, while others may require cross-pollination to bear fruit. Understanding the fruiting timeline also helps plan your garden's visual appeal across seasons. Incorporating fruit plants with staggered harvest times can ensure that you have both blooms and fruits at various points throughout the year, maintaining visual interest and productivity.

Visual Arrangement: Crafting an Appealing Edible Landscape

The visual arrangement of edible plants plays a crucial role in the overall aesthetic of your balcony garden. When positioning plants, consider their individual characteristics and how they interact visually. Creating height variations using plant stands or hanging planters can add dimension and allow lower-growing plants to receive sufficient light. Edible flowers, such as nasturtiums or calendula, can be interspersed among vegetables and herbs to introduce vibrant colors and attract beneficial insects, enhancing the garden's beauty and health.

Furthermore, attractive containers can complement the plants they house. Choose pots in colors and materials that harmonize with the surrounding environment and the plants' hues. Consistency in pot style or color can unify the space while varying the sizes and heights of containers adds visual interest. Regular grooming and harvesting of edible plants encourage healthier growth and maintain the tidy appearance of your garden, ensuring that it remains an inviting and beautiful space on your balcony.

By carefully selecting and arranging attractive and productive edible plants, you can create a garden that serves as a source of culinary inspiration and visual delight. This dual-purpose approach maximizes the utility of limited urban space and enhances the quality of life by providing a beautiful and bountiful green retreat.

Using Upcycled Materials Creatively

Sustainable Gardening: Embracing Upcycling in Urban Settings

In the context of urban gardening, sustainability is not just a buzzword; it's a practical approach to maximizing resources while minimizing waste. One of the most effective ways to achieve this is by using upcycled materials in your garden. Upcycling, the process of repurposing old or discarded materials into new products of higher quality or value, is a cornerstone of sustainable gardening. It allows you to reduce waste, save money, and inject personal style and creativity into your garden.

For urban dwellers, upcycled materials can be sourced from various places, including local thrift stores, recycling bins, or even your own home. Old containers that might otherwise end up in landfill, such as plastic bottles, wooden crates, or even worn-out furniture, can be transformed into unique, eco-friendly plant containers. This practice supports environmental sustainability by reducing waste and adds a layer of unique charm and character to your garden that cannot be replicated with store-bought products. Moreover, by incorporating upcycled materials, you actively contribute to a cycle of reuse that supports broader environmental goals, such as reducing landfill use and minimizing the carbon footprint associated with producing new garden containers and accessories.

Creative Containers: Transforming Everyday Objects into Plant Holders

The transformation of everyday objects into plant containers is a testament to the versatility and potential of upcycled materials. Virtually any object that can hold soil and allow drainage can be converted into a plant holder. For instance, old teapots, boots, or kitchen colanders can become quirky and eye-catching plant containers. To convert these items into suitable plant homes, ensure they have adequate drainage (holes can be drilled if necessary) and are cleaned to remove harmful residues.

Consider the object's material when deciding which plants to place in it. Metal containers, for example, can conduct heat and may be better suited to heat-tolerant plants if exposed to direct sunlight. Similarly, porous materials like untreated wood can offer good moisture retention but may require a protective lining to prevent rot. The choice of plants can also play into the character of the container; for instance, succulents in an old computer monitor can create a playful contrast between technology and nature. By selecting containers that reflect your personal style and considering their interactions with plant choices, you create a sustainable garden that reflects your personality and aesthetic preferences.

DIY Decor: Crafting Garden Accessories from Upcycled Materials

Beyond containers, upcycled materials can be used to create a variety of garden accessories that enhance the functionality and appearance of your urban garden. Simple DIY projects might include creating labels for your plants from painted stones or crafting a watering can from an old milk jug. These projects add a personal touch to your garden and promote a sustainable lifestyle by repurposing materials that would otherwise be discarded.

More ambitious DIY decor projects can involve larger-scale transformations. Pallets, for example, can be converted into vertical garden frames, ladder shelves for plants, or even rustic benches for garden seating. The use of such materials not only saves money but also gives new life to objects that have outlived their original purpose. Each project can be tailored to fit your urban garden's specific constraints and style, ensuring that every element is functional and visually appealing. Learn more about upcycling materials, and other DIY projects, in Chapter 10 starting on page 205.

Resourcefulness: Cultivating Creativity and Efficiency in Garden Design

Adopting a mindset of resourcefulness is key to successful upcycling and sustainable gardening. This approach involves seeing potential in unexpected places and imagining new uses for old items. It encourages continuous learning and adaptation, qualities that are invaluable in urban gardening, where space and resources can be limited. By embracing creativity in the use of upcycled materials, you not only enhance the sustainability of your garden but also develop skills and knowledge that can be applied across various aspects of life.

Resourcefulness in gardening also involves proactively seeking out materials that can be upcycled and being willing to experiment with different configurations and uses. Networking with other gardeners, participating in community exchanges, or even exploring online platforms for inspiration can provide new ideas and resources for upcycling projects. Each act of resourcefulness not only contributes to a more sustainable garden but also fosters a sense of community and shared purpose among urban gardeners, who together can significantly impact sustainability in their environments.

By integrating upcycled materials into your garden design through creative containers, DIY decor, and a resourceful approach, you contribute to a sustainable gardening practice that benefits both the environment and your community. This method of gardening not only provides a practical solution to the challenges of urban gardening but also enriches your gardening experience, making each plant and decor piece a testament to both sustainability and creativity.

The Role of Mulching in Container Gardening

Mulching is a critical yet often overlooked aspect of container gardening that offers numerous benefits to urban gardeners. Primarily, mulch retains moisture in the soil, which is particularly vital in the confined space of a container where soil can dry out rapidly. By maintaining a layer of mulch on top of the soil, evaporation is significantly reduced, and the need for frequent watering decreases, a boon for the busy urban gardener. This moisture retention is crucial during hot weather when water evaporates quickly and plants risk dehydration. Additionally, mulch helps suppress weed growth, which is essential for maintaining a neat and manageable container garden. Weeds not only detract from the aesthetic appeal of your garden but also compete with your plants for vital resources such as nutrients, water, and light. By inhibiting weed germination and growth, mulch ensures that your plants remain the focal point of your garden efforts.

The choice of mulch can vary widely, each type offering unique benefits and considerations. Organic mulches, such as bark chips, straw, and leaf mold, are popular choices for container gardens. These materials break down over time, adding organic matter to the soil and improving its structure and fertility. This gradual decomposition feeds the soil microorganisms, which in turn nourish the plants. Inorganic mulches, including pebbles, gravel, and rubber chips, do not enrich the soil but are more permanent, offering a low-maintenance solution that does not need to be replenished regularly. These materials are particularly suited for decorative purposes or for plants that prefer dry conditions, as they minimize soil moisture retention.

Applying mulch to container plants requires a careful approach to avoid common pitfalls. It is vital to ensure that the mulch does not come into direct contact with the plant stems or leaves, as this can cause rot or fungal infections. Clear space around the plant base will prevent moisture buildup on the plant itself while still allowing the soil to benefit from the moisture-conserving and weed-suppressing properties of the mulch. The thickness of the mulch layer is also crucial; a layer of one to two inches is generally sufficient to suppress weeds and retain moisture without risking soil oxygen deprivation. It's important to apply mulch to moist soil to lock in the moisture and to check periodically that the mulch has not compacted over time, which can prevent water from penetrating the soil.

In addition to its practical benefits, mulching can enhance your container garden's visual appeal. Various colors and textures are available, and mulch can be selected to complement both the plants and the containers they reside in. Dark mulches can make the colors of flowers and foliage pop, while lighter mulches can brighten shady corners and give your garden a clean look. The aesthetic versatility of mulch allows it to be an integral part of the garden design, contributing to the overall visual harmony and thematic styling of your space.

Mulching is a multifaceted practice supporting container gardens' health and beauty. It offers a practical solution to the challenges of urban gardening by conserving water and suppressing weeds while enhancing the soil's fertility and the garden's aesthetic appeal. By choosing the appropriate type of mulch and applying it correctly, you can greatly improve the conditions of your container garden, making it both more productive and more pleasing to the eye.

As we conclude this exploration of mulching and its integral role in container gardening, it's clear that this simple yet effective practice is essential for optimizing the health and appearance of your urban garden. From moisture retention and weed suppression to aesthetic enhancement, the benefits of mulching are wide-ranging. As we transition into the next chapter, we will delve into further techniques and strategies to enhance the productivity and sustainability of your container garden, continuing to expand your capabilities and enjoyment as an urban gardener.

Benefits of Using Mulch

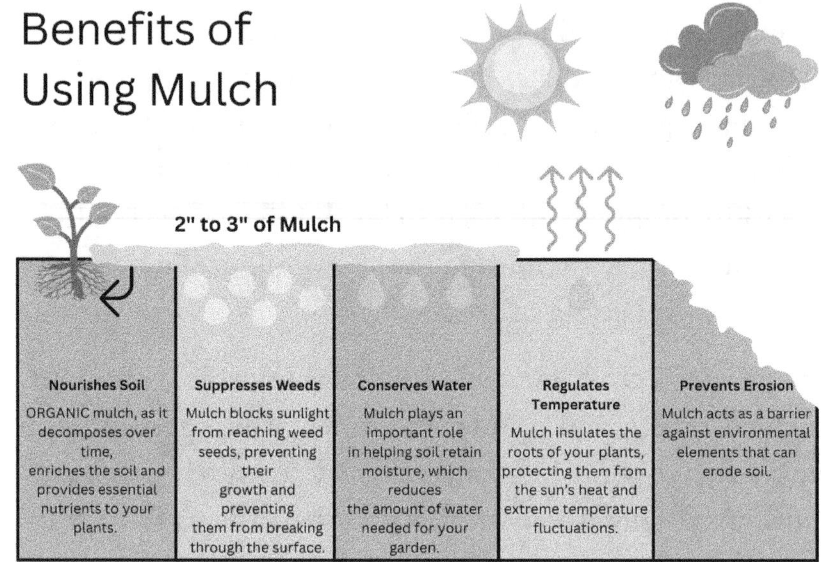

Detail of the many benefits of using mulch

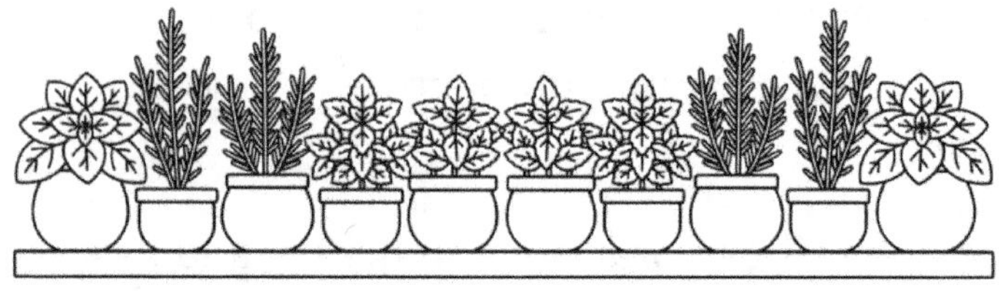

Key Chapter 2 Takeaways:

- Sketch or visualize your layout before placing containers, using balance, contrast, repetition, and scale to keep the space cohesive.

- Plan for mature plant size and growth habit now to avoid overcrowding, poor airflow, and light blockage later.

- Build visual depth using height changes (stands, shelves, trellises, hanging elements) without blocking key light sources.

- Choose a color strategy (calming, energizing, seasonal rotation, foliage-forward, or themed) that matches your space and maintenance level.

- Use vertical gardening, edible ornamentals, upcycled containers, and mulch to improve space efficiency, sustainability, moisture retention, and overall polish.

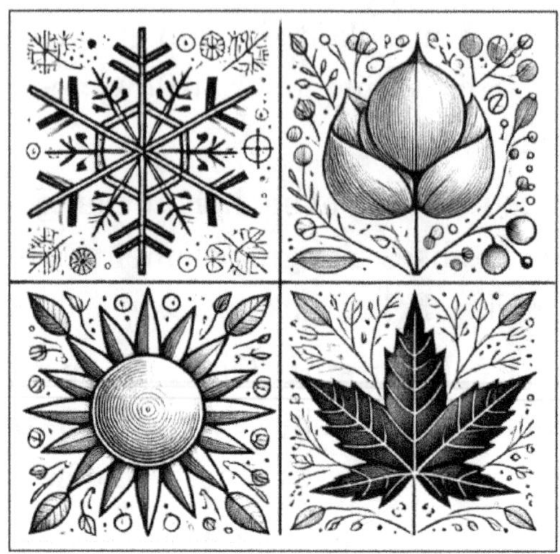

Chapter 3: Seasonal Planning and Plant Selection

In the realm of urban gardening, understanding the ebb and flow of seasons and adapting your garden accordingly isn't just a skill, it's an art. This chapter delves into the critical aspects of seasonal planning and plant selection, tailored specifically for the urban gardener with limited space. Here, you will learn to navigate the complexities of microclimates and hardiness zones, enhancing your ability to make informed decisions about plant selection that align with the unique environmental conditions of your urban garden. This knowledge is not merely functional; it empowers you to extend the thriving period of your garden, ensuring a vibrant green space throughout the year.

Understanding Hardiness Zones and Microclimates

Geographical Impact on Plant Selection and Gardening Timelines

Hardiness zones, a geographic categorization created to denote where various perennial plants can thrive based on minimum winter temperatures, are essential for any gardener to understand. These zones help predict which plants can survive your local winter conditions. This knowledge is crucial for urban gardeners in selecting plants that will survive and flourish in their specific locales. By consulting the USDA Hardiness Zone Map (https://planthardiness.ars.usda.gov), you can identify your specific zone and use this as a guideline to select appropriate plants for your climate. This ensures that your gardening efforts are both efficient and effective, minimizing plant loss due to incompatible climate conditions and maximizing the health and productivity of your garden.

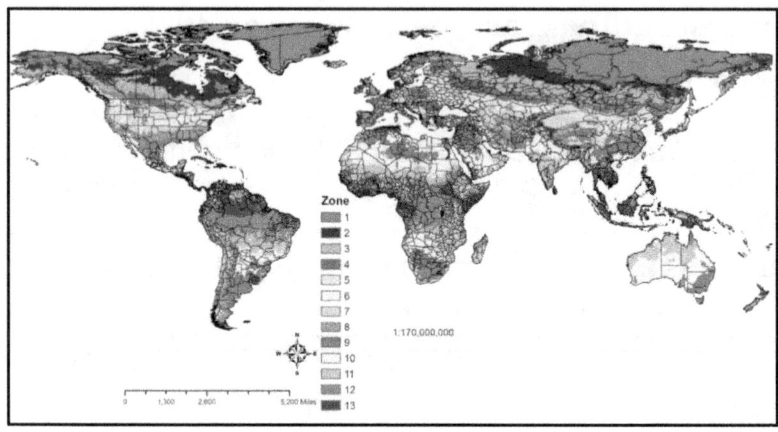

Global Plant Hardiness Zones

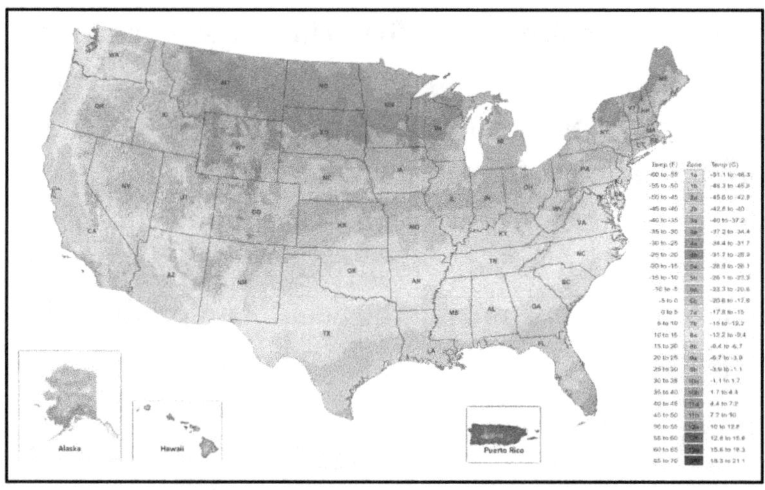

United States Plant Hardiness Zones

Microclimate Identification: Optimizing Plant Placement

Microclimates are small areas within your gardening space where climatic conditions differ from the surrounding areas. In an urban setting, these can be influenced by factors such as proximity to buildings (which can block sunlight or trap heat), ground surfaces (like concrete that may radiate heat), and elevation changes (which can alter wind exposure and temperature). Identifying these microclimates is pivotal for the strategic placement of plants. For instance, a corner that receives less sunlight and is shielded from wind might be ideal for shade-loving plants, while a sunnier, more exposed area could be perfect for sun-thriving varieties. Understanding these subtle nuances within your garden's microclimates allows for a tailored approach to planting, which can significantly boost your garden's overall health and yield.

Adaptation Strategies: Matching Plants to Your Urban Environment

Adapting your plant choices to the specific conditions of your hardiness zone and identifying microclimates optimizes survival and enhances growth and productivity. If your balcony or garden space falls within a cooler, windier zone, selecting plants that are known for their hardiness in cooler temperatures and resistance to wind stress, such as certain conifers or hardy shrubs, will be more successful. Conversely, if your urban space is warmer, leveraging the heat by growing heat-tolerant and drought-resistant plants can turn a potential gardening challenge into a flourishing opportunity. This strategic adaptation to local conditions is what sets successful urban gardens apart.

Resource Utilization: Leveraging Local Expertise and Technology

Maximizing your garden's success involves utilizing every resource at your disposal. Engage with local gardening centers or extension services, which can provide valuable insights into the best plants for your area's specific hardiness zone and microclimates. These local resources often offer plant varieties optimized for the regional climate, which can significantly increase your garden's success rate.

Additionally, technology can play a crucial role in helping you manage your garden more effectively. Various gardening apps provide localized weather updates, reminders for plant care, and even advice on plant selection based on your climate zone. These tools can help you make informed decisions and adapt your garden planning to real-time environmental conditions, ensuring that your urban garden remains vibrant and productive through changing seasons.

Spring: Awakening Your Garden

Spring brings with it the promise of renewal, an ideal time for urban gardeners to reinvigorate their gardens. The first step in this seasonal shift is a thorough assessment and cleanup of your garden containers, which have likely endured the harshness of winter. This process involves examining each container for damage, such as cracks or deterioration, that could impact their functionality. It's also a crucial period to clear out any debris, dead plants, or remnants of last season's growth that could harbor pests or diseases. Cleaning your containers is not merely about aesthetics; it removes potential threats that could compromise plant health in the upcoming seasons. Use a diluted bleach solution (9 parts water to 1 part bleach), vinegar solution (4 parts water to 1 part vinegar), or a natural disinfectant to cleanse the containers, ensuring they are ready to support new growth. This foundational cleanliness sets the stage for a healthy growing environment, which is crucial for the success of your spring garden.

Following the cleanup, your attention should shift to preparing the garden for new plantings. This preparation involves several key tasks, each contributing to creating a conducive growing environment. Begin with refreshing or replacing the soil in your containers. Over the past seasons, the soil in your containers has likely become compacted and nutrient depleted. Replacing or enhancing the soil with fresh, high-quality potting mix can provide a nutrient-rich base for new plantings. Consider mixing in well-composted organic matter, which not only improves soil texture and fertility but also enhances its water-holding capacity, which is vital for plant health during the fluctuating temperatures of spring.

When choosing what to plant in early spring, opt for species known for their resilience to cool temperatures. Pansies, for example, are vibrant, colorful, and cold-tolerant, making them a perfect choice for early planting. Similarly, vegetables like spinach and lettuce can tolerate cooler temperatures and be sown directly into refreshed container soil. These early starters capitalize on the cool weather and provide a gratifying early harvest, boosting your morale for the gardening season ahead.

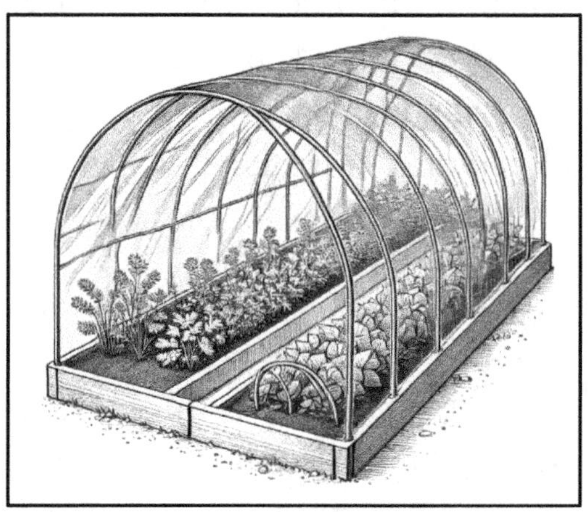

Example of a row cover

Spring is also a time when late frosts can threaten tender new growth, necessitating measures for frost protection. Techniques such as covering plants with floating row covers or bringing portable containers indoors during unusually cold nights can shield your sensitive plants from frost damage. These protective measures are especially important for safeguarding young seedlings, which are particularly vulnerable to temperature fluctuations. Implementing such strategies not only helps extend the growing season but also ensures that your efforts in planting and maintenance do not go to waste due to unexpected frost.

Maintaining the health of your garden as it emerges from winter into the brisk beginnings of spring is pivotal. Regularly check your plants for signs of stress or disease and respond promptly to any issues. Early spring is also an opportune time to start a routine plant-feeding program. A balanced, slow-release fertilizer can provide a steady supply of nutrients, supporting the initial stages of growth and development. Watering should also be adjusted during this time; while the soil should remain moist, be wary of overwatering, as cool spring weather can slow the drying of soil, increasing the risk of root rot.

By assessing and preparing your garden in early spring, refreshing the soil, choosing the right plants for early planting, protecting them from late frosts, and maintaining their health through vigilant care, you set the stage for a thriving garden that will flourish throughout the growing season. This proactive approach in the early weeks of spring revitalizes your garden and renews your connection with nature as you nurture and watch your plants grow.

Summer: Maintaining Vibrance and Productivity

As the zenith of the growing season, summer presents opportunities and challenges for the urban gardener. Your garden, now in full bloom and vigor, requires attentive care to maintain its productivity and visual appeal during the warmer months. This period is crucial for nurturing heat-loving plants, adjusting watering schedules to combat the intense sun, vigilantly guarding against pests, and considering midsummer planting for continued harvests.

Heat-Loving Plants: Thriving in Summer Warmth

Certain plants not only withstand the summer heat but thrive in it. These varieties are particularly suited to the sweltering days of July and August, making them ideal for urban gardens exposed to full sun. Consider species such as tomatoes, peppers, eggplants, and zucchini, which are well-known for their preference for warmer weather. These plants benefit from consistent heat, significantly enhancing their growth and fruiting potential. Similarly, flowers like marigolds, petunias, and zinnias add a splash of color to your garden while thriving in hot conditions.

Caring for these heat-loving plants goes beyond mere survival; it involves strategies to optimize their growth. Firstly, ensure they are planted in well-draining soil to prevent root rot from excessive watering. Adding a layer of mulch can help retain soil moisture and keep the roots cool. Regular feeding is crucial, as the rapid growth of these plants in summer can deplete nutrients quickly. Use a balanced fertilizer to promote healthy foliage and abundant fruiting or blooming. Additionally, providing some form of shade during the hottest part of the day can prevent scorching and stress, particularly for younger plants that have not yet fully established their heat tolerance.

Watering Adjustments: Adapting to Increased Heat

The rise in temperatures during summer months results in faster water evaporation from the soil, necessitating more frequent watering to keep plants hydrated. However, this does not simply mean watering more often but watering more effectively. Early morning is the ideal time for watering, as it allows water to reach deep into the soil before the day's heat accelerates evaporation. If watering in the evening, ensure it is early enough so that the foliage can dry before nightfall, reducing the risk of fungal diseases.

Check moisture levels daily in containers, which can heat up more quickly than ground soil. Containers with moisture-retaining polymers mixed into the soil can help buffer against rapid drying. Consider setting up a drip irrigation system (explained in Chapter 7, section 4) for a steady, regulated supply of water that meets plants' needs without wastage. Such systems are particularly beneficial in urban settings where daily hand-watering may not be feasible.

Pest Vigilance: Guarding Against Summer Invaders

Summer also invites a host of garden pests that can threaten the health and productivity of your plants. Common culprits include aphids, spider mites, and whiteflies, which are attracted to stressed plants in dry, hot conditions. Regular inspections of your plants are critical; pay special attention to the undersides of leaves where pests often congregate. Implementing an integrated pest management (IPM) approach can effectively control these pests. This might include introducing beneficial insects, such as ladybugs, which prey on aphids, or applying neem oil, an organic pesticide that is safe for beneficial insects and humans.

Additionally, maintaining strong plant health is your first defense against pests. Stressed plants are more susceptible to pest infestations, whether from under-watering, overwatering, or nutrient deficiencies. Ensuring your plants are well cared for and not stressed by their environment reduces the likelihood of severe pest problems.

Midsummer Planting: Extending the Harvest

Midsummer offers an opportunity to extend your garden's productivity by planting second crops that will mature by late summer or early fall. Fast-growing vegetables like greens (lettuce, spinach) or radishes can be sown directly into the soil now and will benefit from the still-warm soil and cooler late-summer days. Additionally, consider planting herbs such as cilantro or dill, which can bolt (when a plant begins to flower and produce seeds before its ready to harvest) in the heat but will thrive if planted during the slightly cooler part of summer.

This practice of successive planting ensures a continuous supply of produce and optimizes the use of your garden space. As early summer crops finish and are harvested, replenishing the soil and planting new crops can keep your garden vibrant and productive well into the fall. This not only maximizes your yield but also maintains the aesthetic appeal of your garden, as spent and harvested plants are replaced with vigorous new growth.

The summer months demand a vigilant and proactive approach to garden care, emphasizing the need for strategic watering, pest management, and plant selection. By embracing these practices, you ensure that your urban garden survives the summer heat and thrives, providing a lush, productive, and beautiful space during these vibrant months.

Fall: Preparing for the Cooler Months

As the vibrant effusions of summer begin to wane, the cooler, quieter months of fall provide a perfect opportunity for urban gardeners to prepare their spaces for the impending winter. This season is not merely about winding down but involves strategic planning that ensures your garden's sustainability and productivity through fall and beyond. Selecting the right plants for fall planting and harvesting is crucial during this period. Vegetables such as kale, collards, and Brussels sprouts thrive in the cooling temperatures of fall and can be harvested well into the early winter in some climates. These crops benefit from the chill as it enhances their flavors, making them ideal choices for your autumn garden. Additionally, incorporating ornamental plants like chrysanthemums or asters can add splashes of color to your garden as other plants begin to fade.

Fall is also an appropriate time to introduce bulbs such as tulips, daffodils, and alliums, which require a wintering over period underground to bloom in the spring. Planting these bulbs in containers in the fall ensures a vibrant burst of color the following season, rejuvenating your garden after the cold winter months. Moreover, it's essential to consider the microclimate of your gardening space when selecting these plants. Areas that retain more warmth or are shielded from harsh winds can support a wider variety of fall crops and ornamentals, potentially extending their growing and blooming period further into the winter.

The transition to cooler weather also signifies the need for a thorough garden cleanup. Removing spent summer crops and any plant debris is vital to preventing the proliferation of pests and diseases over the winter. This cleanup should be meticulous, involving pruning dead or dying branches from perennial plants and carefully inspecting all plants for signs of disease or infestation. Any diseased plant material should be discarded far from your garden area to prevent the spread of pathogens. This process helps maintain the health of your garden and prepares the space for new plantings. Tidying your garden in the fall can be a meditative process, allowing you to reflect on the past season's successes while preparing for the future.

Mulching for Protection

Mulching in fall plays a critical role in protecting your plants during the cooler months. Organic mulches such as straw, shredded leaves, or wood chips can be applied to your container plants to insulate the soil against sudden temperature drops that are common in late fall. This insulation helps maintain a consistent soil temperature, protecting roots from freeze-thaw cycles that can heave and damage them. Also, mulch helps retain soil moisture, as dry winter winds can quickly dehydrate soil. Apply a thick layer of mulch, approximately two to three inches, around your plants, leaving some space around the stem bases to prevent moisture accumulation, which could lead to rot.

Mulch can be aesthetically pleasing, particularly in containers, giving your garden a tidy, cared-for look while performing an essential protective function. As the organic mulches slowly decompose, they contribute to the soil's nutrient content, enhancing its fertility and structure for the next planting season. This dual role of mulch, both protective and nourishing, makes it an indispensable component of fall gardening practices.

Extending the Season

Extending the growing season into the early fall can significantly increase your garden's yield and allow you to enjoy fresh produce for longer. Techniques such as using cold frames or floating row covers can create slightly warmer microenvironments than the external climate, protecting plants from early frosts. Cold frames, which can be built from old windows or clear plastic sheeting, trap sunlight during the day, keeping plants warm as temperatures drop at night. Floating row covers, made from lightweight fabric, can be draped over plants to provide a similar warming effect while allowing light and moisture to reach the plants.

Another strategy involves selecting late-maturing varieties of vegetables or those with shorter growing cycles that can be harvested before the first frost. For instance, fast-growing leafy greens like spinach or mustard can be sown in late summer and harvested throughout the fall. Similarly, root vegetables like carrots and beets can be left in the soil and harvested as needed, their underground position providing some natural protection against mild frosts. By implementing these strategies, you not only maximize your garden's productivity but also enhance your enjoyment of it, extending the pleasures of gardening later into the year.

Each step taken in fall, from selecting the right plants and cleaning up your garden to applying mulch and extending the season, prepares your urban garden for the colder months ahead while maximizing its beauty and bounty. These efforts ensure that your garden remains a source of joy and nourishment, reflecting the careful planning and love invested throughout the year. As you wrap up these fall activities, your garden stands ready, robust, and resilient, poised to weather the winter and burst forth anew in the spring.

Winter: Keeping Your Garden Alive

Winter presents a unique set of challenges and opportunities for the urban gardener. Despite the cold and often harsh conditions, it's possible to maintain a lively container garden that not only survives but thrives during these months. A key strategy involves selecting winter-hardy plants that are well-suited to colder temperatures. Varieties such as winter kale, evergreen shrubs, and ornamental cabbages endure the winter chill and add a splash of color and life to your urban space when most other plants have succumbed to the frost. These plants have adapted to the cold and can often manage with the light levels available during shorter days, making them perfect for brightening up a dreary winter balcony or patio.

Equally important is the care of plants that are not naturally winter hardy. Moving delicate plants indoors during the coldest months offers a practical solution for many urban gardeners. Before transitioning plants indoors, it is crucial to consider the environmental differences they will encounter. Indoor environments typically offer warmer temperatures but can have lower humidity levels and less natural light than outdoors. Gradually acclimatizing your plants to these new conditions can prevent shock, allowing them to adjust without significant stress. This might involve placing them in a sheltered but cool area of your home where they receive ample indirect light. Additionally, consider the space's humidity and, if necessary, use a humidifier or place water trays near heating sources to increase moisture levels in the air, which helps maintain the health of the plants.

Protecting your outdoor plants from frost is another vital winter task. Techniques such as wrapping pots in burlap or bubble wrap can insulate roots from freezing temperatures. This is particularly important for perennial plants in containers, as their roots are more exposed to cold than those planted in the ground. For added protection, moving pots against the house or under a shelter can shield them from harsh winds and provide a slightly warmer microclimate. Elevated platforms can prevent the cold from seeping into pots from frozen ground surfaces, further insulating plant roots. These protective measures extend the life of your plants through the winter and prepare them for successful growth in the spring.

Winter also provides an invaluable opportunity for planning the upcoming gardening season. This downtime can be used to reflect on the past year's successes and challenges, allowing you to strategize for the year ahead. Researching new plant varieties, planning garden layouts, and even starting some plants indoors can get a head start on the spring gardening season. Consider browsing gardening catalogs or websites to find new and exciting plant species that might become the next great addition to your urban garden. Planning in winter allows you to order seeds and bulbs ahead of time, ensuring that you are ready to plant as soon as the weather permits.

This period of relative garden inactivity is an excellent time to perform maintenance on gardening tools and containers Learn more about tool maintenance in Chapter 9 on page 191. Cleaning, sharpening, and oiling tools extend their life and make gardening more effective and enjoyable. Inspecting containers for cracks or wear and cleaning them to remove soil residues and potential pathogens ensures that your garden infrastructure is in top condition for spring planting. These preparatory activities might not be as glamorous as planting or harvesting, but they are crucial for maintaining the functionality and aesthetics of your garden, setting a solid foundation for the lush growth to come with the return of spring.

Year-Round Edibles for Your Container Garden

Perennial Edibles: Sustaining Your Garden Across Seasons

Incorporating perennial edibles into your urban container garden offers a sustainable approach to cultivating food that can provide yields year after year with proper care. Unlike annuals, which complete their life cycle in one growing season, perennials return each season, offering multiple harvests for a one-time planting effort. This enduring presence makes them particularly suitable for gardeners looking for long-term gardening solutions in limited spaces. For instance, herbs such as rosemary, thyme, and sage are excellent perennial choices for containers, offering culinary benefits and enduring greenery and pleasant aromas. Additionally, some vegetables act as perennials in certain climates. Asparagus, for example, once established, can produce tender shoots each spring for many years. Rhubarb is another robust plant known for its tangy stalks that can be harvested each year in late spring to early summer.

The key to successful perennial gardening in containers lies in choosing the right varieties that can adapt to the confined space and potentially less-than-ideal growing conditions of urban settings. Ensuring that the container is large enough to accommodate the plant's mature size and root system and that the soil is well-nourished and well-draining to support its long-term growth is crucial. Moreover, perennial plants often require less regular replanting but might need annual pruning or division to keep them healthy and productive. Once established, this makes them a less labor-intensive option, suitable for urban gardeners who appreciate both the practical and aesthetic benefits of green spaces but might have limited time for garden maintenance.

Continuous Harvesting: Maximizing Garden Output

Continuous harvesting is a technique designed to extend the production period of your garden, ensuring a steady supply of fresh produce. This approach involves strategic planting and harvesting methods that keep the garden productive beyond the typical growing season. Succession planting is one such method, where you stagger the planting of certain crops at intervals throughout the season. For example, planting a new batch of lettuce seeds every two weeks results in a continuous supply of fresh lettuce rather than a single, large harvest that might not be consumed quickly. This method can be particularly beneficial for urban gardeners with limited space, as it maximizes the use of the garden area and extends the harvest period over many months.

Another aspect of continuous harvesting involves selecting varieties of plants that mature at different times, which can be particularly effective for crops like tomatoes or peppers. Choosing early, mid-season and late-ripening varieties allows you to enjoy fresh produce from early summer into late fall. Implementing a cut-and-come-again approach for leafy greens such as spinach and Swiss chard enables multiple harvests from the same plant. By harvesting only the outer leaves and allowing the younger inner leaves to mature, you can sustain a plant's productivity significantly longer than if you harvested it all at once.

Indoor Herb Gardens: Cultivating Flavors Year-Round

Maintaining an indoor herb garden allows you to enjoy fresh herbs regardless of the season, making it an excellent option for urban dwellers who may not have access to outdoor space during the colder months. Herbs such as basil, cilantro, parsley, and chives are well-suited to indoor conditions if they receive sufficient light. Ideally, a south-facing window offering at least six hours of sunlight daily is perfect, but if natural light is insufficient, grow lights can provide the necessary light levels.

When setting up an indoor herb garden, consider using a high-quality potting mix and ensure proper drainage to avoid waterlogged soil, which can lead to root rot. Regular harvesting encourages the plants to produce new growth, keeping them lush and productive. Additionally, be mindful of the indoor environment. Herbs prefer a relatively humid atmosphere, which might require the use of a humidifier in dry indoor conditions, especially during winter when heating systems are in use. By managing these factors, your indoor herb garden can thrive, providing fresh flavors and a touch of greenery to your living space year-round.

Cold-Frame Gardening: Extending the Growing Season

Cold frames, essentially mini greenhouses, offer a practical solution for extending the growing season of edibles, especially in climates with colder winters. Constructed from transparent material set over a sturdy frame, cold frames trap solar heat and insulate plants from cold weather, allowing you to start your spring planting earlier and extend the fall growing season later than would be possible outdoors. This can be particularly beneficial for growing vegetables like carrots, beets, and leafy greens, which can tolerate lower temperatures but may need protection from frost and harsh winds.

Using a cold frame can be as simple as placing it over existing garden containers or directly onto a garden bed. Monitoring the temperature inside the cold frame is vital, as sunny days can quickly lead to overheating, even in cold weather. Ventilating the cold frame by opening the top during warm days and closing it at night or when temperatures drop prevents temperature extremes that could damage plants. With proper management, a cold frame can turn a seasonal garden into a nearly year-round venture, significantly boosting the productivity and efficiency of your urban gardening efforts.

This exploration of year-round edibles for your container garden underscores the adaptability and resilience of urban gardening practices. By integrating perennial plants, employing continuous harvesting techniques, maintaining indoor herb gardens, and utilizing cold frames, you can enjoy fresh produce throughout the year, regardless of your urban setting's traditional growing seasons. These strategies enhance your garden's yield and aesthetic appeal and contribute to a sustainable lifestyle, epitomizing the profound connection between nature and urban life. As you continue cultivating your garden, these practices will prove invaluable, ensuring that your green space remains vibrant and productive, whatever the season.

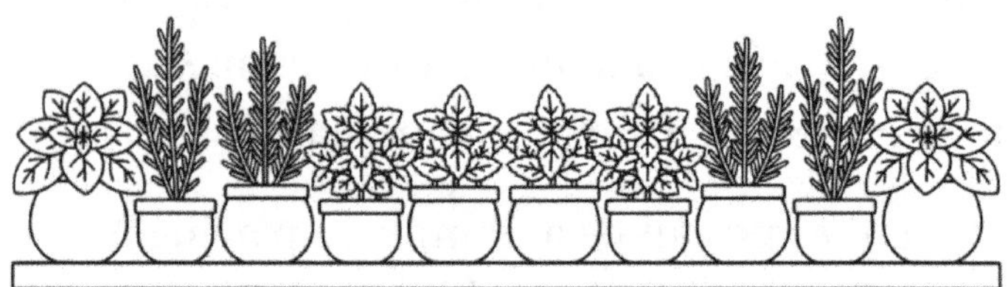

Key Chapter 3 Takeaways:

- Use your USDA hardiness zone as a baseline for plant selection, then fine-tune choices based on your balcony's microclimates (sun, wind, heat, shelter).

- Start each spring with a simple reset: inspect containers, clean/disinfect, refresh soil, and choose cool-tolerant early plants while preparing for late frosts.

- In summer, protect productivity by adjusting watering (especially in containers), using mulch, monitoring moisture daily, and watching for pests early.

- In fall, focus on cleanup, cold-tolerant planting, and insulation (mulch, covers, cold frames) to prevent winter carryover problems.

- Keep the garden going year-round by combining winter-hardy choices, indoor transitions for tender plants, container insulation, and planning tools like succession planting and indoor herbs.

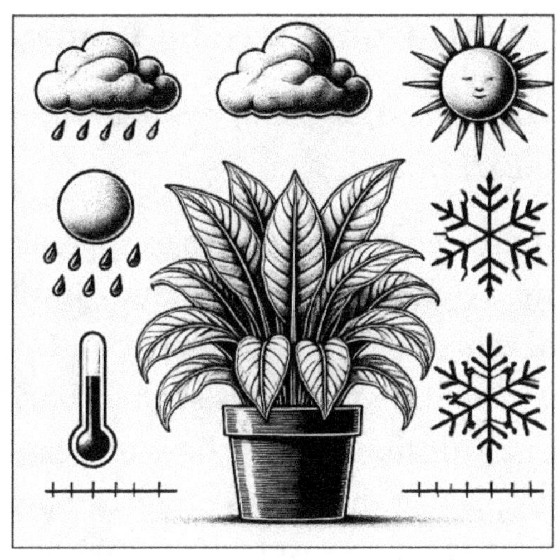

Chapter 4: Overcoming Seasonal Challenges

Navigating the changing of seasons presents a spectrum of challenges and opportunities for urban gardeners. Each season ushers in a unique set of environmental conditions that can either propel your garden to flourish or pose significant threats to its vitality. Understanding how to manage these seasonal dynamics effectively is crucial, particularly when it comes to protecting your plants from extreme temperatures. This chapter delves into sophisticated strategies designed to shield your garden from the harsh realities of temperature fluctuations, ensuring that your green sanctuary remains robust and vibrant throughout the year.

Protecting Plants from Extreme Temperatures

Insulation Techniques: Crafting a Shield Against Temperature Extremes

Extreme hot and cold temperatures can wreak havoc on urban gardens. To safeguard your plants, implementing effective insulation techniques is essential. During the cold months, insulating materials such as burlap, bubble wrap, or specially designed plant blankets can be wrapped around pots to protect the roots from freezing. This is particularly crucial for perennial plants whose root systems may be vulnerable to frost heaving, a condition where roots are pushed out of the soil due to the natural freeze-thaw cycle, damaging or killing the plant.

Consider elevating your containers off the cold ground on wooden or foam blocks for added protection. This creates an air barrier that minimizes heat transfer from the pot to the cold ground or vice versa. Additionally, grouping your plants together can help create a microclimate that slightly raises the temperature among the plants, providing collective insulation. However, ensure there is sufficient air circulation to prevent moisture buildup, which could lead to fungal diseases.

Heat can be just as detrimental when temperatures soar, causing overheating and sunburn in plants. To combat this, white or reflective pot covers can be used to deflect sunlight and reduce heat absorption. Alternatively, materials such as shade cloth can be draped over sensitive plants during the hottest part of the day to reduce temperature stress. Monitoring the weather and providing shade before the temperatures peak is crucial, as preventative measures are more effective than trying to alleviate stress after the fact.

Shade Solutions: Preventing Overheating and Sunburn

The strategic use of shade can dramatically reduce the thermal stress on your plants during hot months. Installing temporary shade structures such as canopies or retractable shades can provide much-needed relief from the intense midday sun. These structures should be positioned to cast shade during the peak sunlight hours while allowing for morning and late afternoon sun, which is less intense and beneficial for plant growth.

For a more natural solution, consider using taller plants or trellised vines to shade smaller, more vulnerable species. This enhances the aesthetic appeal of your garden and promotes biodiversity. However, it's important to plan your garden layout to optimize light exposure for all plants, ensuring that the shading plants do not block essential sunlight from the sun-sensitive species.

Temperature Monitoring: Harnessing Technology to Guard Against Extremes

Technology plays a pivotal role in managing environmental conditions in the modern urban garden. Utilizing digital thermometers or temperature sensors can provide real-time data on the microclimates within your garden. These devices can be linked to smartphone apps that alert you when temperature thresholds are exceeded, allowing timely interventions.

Consider installing a weather station in your garden for a more interactive approach. This device can measure temperature, humidity, light levels, and wind speed, offering a comprehensive overview of your garden's climate. This information can be crucial in making informed decisions about plant care, particularly when dealing with fragile or temperature-sensitive plants.

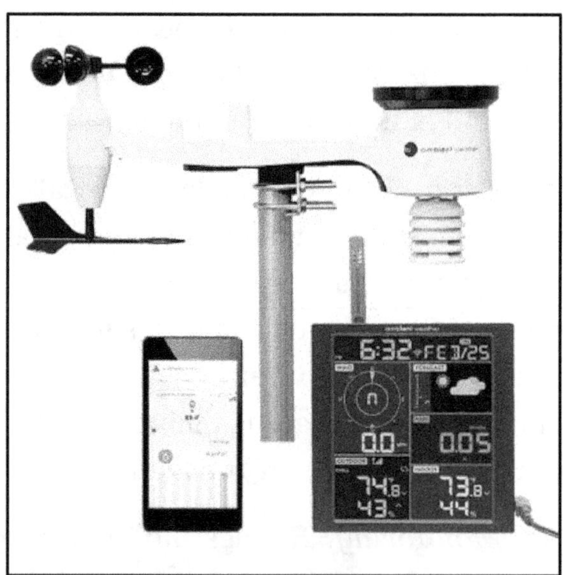

Weather station

Plant Selection: Choosing the Right Plants for Your Microclimate

Selecting naturally adapted plants to withstand local temperature extremes is perhaps the most effective strategy to ensure garden resilience. Research plants that are native to or thrive in climates similar to yours. For instance, in areas with hot summers, opt for drought-resistant plants such as sedum or lavender, which are well-adapted to survive with minimal water and high heat. In cooler climates, look for frost-tolerant plants like kale or pansies, which can survive a light frost.

Consulting with local nurseries or gardening communities can provide insights into the best plants for your specific conditions. These resources often have years of experience in plant performance in your area and can recommend varieties that have proven successful in local urban gardens.

Research your area's plant hardiness zone to assist you in selecting appropriate plants for your garden. This map categorizes geographical areas based on their minimum and maximum temperature ranges, providing a visual guide to understanding the climatic conditions prevalent in your region. By referring to this map, you can make informed decisions about plant selection that align with the thermal characteristics of your local environment, enhancing your garden's ability to thrive in the face of temperature extremes.

Managing Sunlight Variations Throughout the Year

Adjustable Setups: Crafting Dynamic Garden Environments

As the sun takes its varied path through the seasons, the amount of sunlight your garden receives can fluctuate dramatically, impacting the vitality of your plants. Adjustable garden setups are essential to mitigate these changes and provide your plants with the optimal light conditions they require throughout the year. One effective strategy involves the use of mobile container platforms. These platforms or carts equipped with casters allow you to move your plants to locations where sunlight is optimal. For example, during the short winter days, you might wheel your plants to a south-facing location where sunlight is maximized. Conversely, in the height of summer, the same plants could be moved to a spot with partial shade to prevent overexposure to harsh midday sun.

Another adjustable setup includes the use of modular garden structures, such as adjustable trellises or retractable shade cloths. These structures can be manipulated to either increase sunlight exposure or provide necessary shade. Adjustable trellises can be repositioned to optimize the angle of sunlight penetration, which is especially beneficial for climbing plants that might otherwise shade each other out. Retractable shade cloths can be drawn during peak sunlight hours to protect sensitive plants from sunburn and then retracted in the late afternoon or on cloudy days to allow maximum light exposure.

These dynamic setups not only enhance plant health by providing optimal light conditions but also increase the flexibility of urban gardening, making it possible to grow a wider variety of plants in a confined space. By observing the growth and health of your plants, you can continually adjust their positioning, ensuring they always receive the right amount of light without being subjected to the stress of inappropriate sun exposure.

Artificial Lighting: Extending Daylight for Indoor and Shaded Gardens

For many urban gardeners, natural light availability remains a limiting factor, particularly in winter months or in heavily shaded areas. In these cases, artificial lighting can provide a vital supplement that keeps your garden thriving. Grow lights, specifically designed to replicate the spectrum of natural sunlight, can support photosynthesis and plant growth in environments where natural light is insufficient. When selecting grow lights, consider the specific needs of your plants; some might require a full-spectrum light, while others might thrive under lights that emit a specific range of the light spectrum.

Installing grow lights involves more than just setting up a bulb above your plants; it requires thoughtful configuration to ensure light is evenly distributed and at the correct intensity. Lights should be placed at a height that covers all plants but does not cause overheating or light burn. Using timers to control the lights can mimic natural day and night cycles, preventing stress that could result from constant exposure. Moreover, the energy efficiency of LED grow lights makes them an ideal choice for prolonged use, minimizing electricity consumption while providing high-intensity, low-heat light.

Reflective Surfaces: Harnessing Light to Enhance Growth

Using reflective surfaces can significantly increase light availability in urban environments, where tall buildings or narrow spaces can limit direct sunlight. Materials such as reflective mulches, garden mirrors, or even pale-colored walls can be strategically placed to reflect additional light onto your plants. Reflective mulches, typically made from metallic plastic, can be spread on the soil around your plants to reflect sunlight upwards, which is particularly beneficial for low-growing plants that taller neighbors might otherwise shade. Mirrors positioned opposite your garden can double the sunlight your plants receive, dramatically improving photosynthesis and plant vigor.

Placing these reflective surfaces requires careful consideration to avoid causing heat spots or focusing light too intensely, which could damage plants. Ideally, reflective materials should be positioned to bounce sunlight evenly across a broad area of your garden, enhancing light without creating overly hot or bright spots. Experimenting with different placements and observing the effects on your plants will help you optimize the use of reflective surfaces to enhance your garden's light environment effectively.

Seasonal Relocation: Optimizing Plant Exposure Throughout the Year

The mobility of container gardens offers a unique advantage in managing light exposure; plants can be relocated to optimize their growth conditions as seasons change. During spring and fall, when the sun is less intense, plants can be positioned to maximize light exposure, perhaps in a clear, unobstructed part of your balcony or along a sunlit windowsill. As the intensity of the summer sun increases, these same plants might benefit from a location that offers afternoon shade, preventing stress and dehydration.

Seasonal relocation also involves adjusting the vertical positioning of plants. Elevating plants on stands or shelves can prevent shading by surrounding structures or other plants and can be particularly beneficial in densely planted areas where light is at a premium. Conversely, lowering plants closer to the ground can provide a cooler environment during hot spells. Regularly assessing your plants' light needs and health will guide these relocation efforts, ensuring that each plant receives its ideal light exposure for healthy growth.

By implementing these strategies, you ensure that your urban garden adapts seamlessly to the changing angles and intensities of sunlight throughout the year. Whether through adjustable setups, the strategic use of reflective surfaces, the supplementing of natural light with artificial options, or the thoughtful seasonal relocation of your plants, you can maintain a vibrant and productive garden that dynamically responds to the natural light environment, maximizing the health and yield of your plants.

Watering Strategies for Every Season

Understanding and adapting to your plants' seasonal water needs is paramount in maintaining a healthy and thriving urban garden. Plant water requirements vary not only among species but also according to seasonal changes in environmental conditions. During the warmer months, evaporation rates increase, and plants typically exhibit higher growth rates, increasing their water needs. Conversely, plant metabolism slows down in colder months, reducing their water requirements. Recognizing these patterns and adjusting your watering practices accordingly is crucial for ensuring plant health and water efficiency.

In spring, as temperatures begin to rise and plants emerge from their winter dormancy, their water needs gradually increase. This is a critical time for young seedlings and newly planted flora, which require consistent moisture to establish strong root systems. Watering during this season should be attentive to providing sufficient moisture without causing waterlogging, as the soil's ability to absorb water increases with the temperature. As you transition into summer, the watering frequency typically needs to increase. The combination of higher temperatures, longer daylight hours, and active plant growth means soil dries out more quickly. During this peak growing season, it's essential to ensure that your plants receive enough water to support their growth without experiencing stress from drought.

However, the approach changes as you enter autumn. This season often brings cooler temperatures and increased precipitation, which can decrease the need for supplemental watering. Additionally, as plant growth slows in preparation for winter, excessive watering can lead to issues such as root rot or fungal growth. Monitoring rainfall and reducing the frequency of watering as the season progresses will help maintain the right moisture levels in the soil. By winter, most plants have entered a dormant state, and their water requirements reach the lowest point. During these months, focus on preventing the soil from completely drying out, while being cautious not to overwater, especially if your containers are in locations that receive less sunlight and have reduced evaporation rates.

Water Conservation: Implementing Sustainable Practices

Incorporating water conservation techniques into your gardening practice is environmentally responsible and essential for maintaining a sustainable urban garden. Rainwater collection systems, such as rain barrels or cisterns, allow you to capture and store rainwater, which can be a significant resource for watering your garden. This method reduces your reliance on municipal water systems and provides your plants with chemical-free water, which can improve their health and growth.

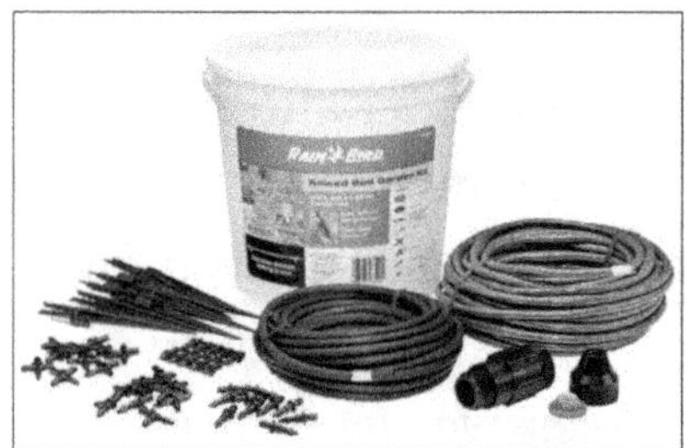
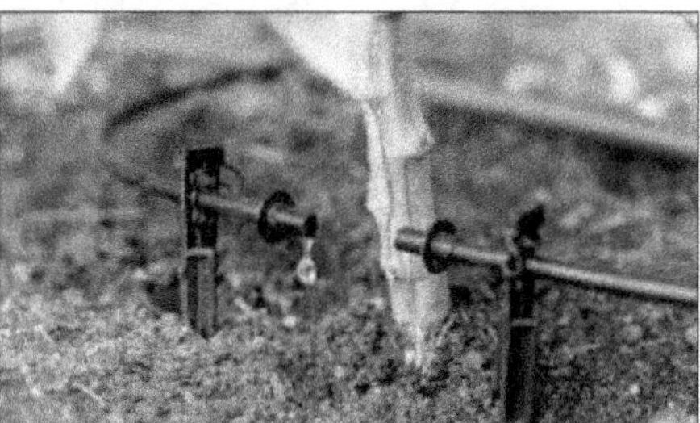

Example of drip irrigation system parts and installed by a plant

Drip irrigation systems offer another efficient solution for urban gardens. These systems deliver water directly to the base of the plant, minimizing waste and reducing evaporation and runoff. Drip irrigation provides a slow, steady supply of water, encouraging deep root growth and helping plants become more drought resistant.

Implementing a drip system can be particularly beneficial during the hot summer months, ensuring that water reaches the roots of plants without being lost to evaporation under the harsh sun.

Monitoring Soil Moisture: Ensuring Optimal Water Levels

Accurately gauging soil moisture is key to preventing overwatering and underwatering, which can stress plants and lead to poor health or death. Soil moisture sensors, available in digital and analog forms, can precisely measure soil humidity, helping you understand when it's time to water. Placing these sensors at the root level in your containers can clearly indicate the moisture available to your plants, allowing you to water more efficiently.

For those who prefer a more hands-on approach, the manual feel test remains a reliable method for assessing soil moisture. By feeling the soil, you can determine its moisture content; dry, crumbly soil indicates a need for water, whereas moist, clumpy soil suggests adequate hydration. Regular checking of soil moisture, especially during seasonal transitions when weather and temperature can fluctuate, supports proactive garden management and promotes plant health.

Mulching for Moisture: A Seasonal Approach to Soil Health

Mulching is an effective technique to conserve soil moisture and ensure your plants have access to water when they need it. Organic mulches, such as wood chips, straw, or leaf mold, help retain moisture by reducing surface evaporation and contribute to soil health as they decompose. In the hot months, a thick layer of mulch can keep the soil cool and moist, reducing the need for frequent watering. As you move into cooler months, mulch plays a vital role by insulating the soil and protecting roots from temperature extremes.

The type and amount of mulch used can vary with the seasons. A lighter mulch layer can warm the soil in spring after the cold winter. Increasing the mulch layer's thickness can help maintain soil moisture and temperature stability as temperatures rise. In autumn, refreshing the mulch can protect plants from sudden temperature drops and provide nutrients for the soil as organic mulches decompose. Adjusting the mulch layers according to seasonal needs enhances your garden's resilience and productivity, ensuring it remains a lush and vibrant space regardless of the time of year.

Pest and Disease Management in Changing Climates

Preventative Measures: Establishing a Foundation for Healthy Plants

The cornerstone of effective pest and disease management in any garden, particularly in urban environments where space is at a premium, lies in implementing robust preventative measures. These strategies are designed not only to combat potential infestations and outbreaks but also to create an environment that inherently discourages pests and diseases from taking hold. One fundamental approach is selecting and cultivating of plant varieties known for their resistance to pests and diseases. Many modern cultivars have been specifically developed to be more resilient against common pathogens and pests, providing an essential layer of defense by reducing the likelihood of outbreaks.

In addition to choosing resistant varieties, ensuring optimal plant health is pivotal in preventing pest and disease problems. Stressed plants are more susceptible to attack, so proper nutrition, adequate watering, and appropriate sun exposure are crucial. This involves regular soil testing to ensure nutrient levels are balanced, adjusting fertilization practices to meet the specific needs of your plants, and ensuring that watering practices promote healthy root development without creating waterlogged conditions that can foster root diseases.

Another preventative strategy involves crop rotation even in a container garden setting. Learn more about container crop rotation in Appendix 1 on page 234. By rotating plants to different containers or areas of your balcony or patio, you can prevent the buildup of soil-borne pests and diseases. Additionally, incorporating companion planting can be beneficial. Certain plant combinations naturally repel pests or enhance each other's growth, which can significantly bolster your garden's defenses against potential infestations.

Early Pest Prevention: Safeguarding Young Plants

Early detection and prevention are key to managing pests effectively, especially when it comes to protecting young, vulnerable plants that are often the most attractive to pests. Learn more about pest prevention in Chapter 10 on page 215. Regularly monitoring your garden is essential; this means inspecting plants closely for any signs of pest activity or disease symptoms such as unusual leaf spots, distorted growth, or insects. Implementing a routine schedule for checking your plants, ideally every few days allows for the early identification of potential issues before they escalate.

For young plants, the use of barriers can be an effective preventive measure. Floating row covers made of lightweight fabric can protect seedlings from pests while still allowing light and air to penetrate, promoting healthy growth. Similarly, the use of insect nets or mesh can prevent flying pests from accessing plants without the use of chemical insecticides. These barriers can be particularly useful during the critical early stages of plant development or when pests are known to be active in your area.

Additionally, fostering a healthy population of beneficial insects such as ladybugs, lacewings, and predatory wasps can help control pest populations naturally. These beneficial insects can be attracted to your garden by planting a diverse array of plants, including those that produce nectar and pollen. Creating a habitat that supports these natural predators provides a dynamic and sustainable pest control method that works continuously throughout the growing season.

Seasonal Pests: Adapting to Seasonal Variabilities

Each season can bring different challenges regarding pests, as many insects and diseases thrive under specific climate conditions. For instance, aphids and spider mites may proliferate in summer's warm, dry conditions, while slugs and snails are more prevalent in spring or fall's cool, moist environment. Recognizing the seasonal patterns of pests in your region is crucial for effective management.

During the spring, preventive applications of organic horticultural oils or insecticidal soaps can be used to manage the early emergence of pests like aphids. These treatments can help reduce populations before they become large enough to cause significant damage. In the summer, vigilance is key as warmer temperatures can accelerate the lifecycle of many pests, increasing their reproduction rates.

As fall approaches, decrease the likelihood of overwintering pests and diseases by cleaning up garden debris and dead plant material, which can harbor pests during winter. This cleanup is crucial to reducing potential outbreaks in the following spring. For pests that are active in the winter, such as certain types of mites or scale insects, the use of dormant oils can provide control without harming dormant plants.

Disease Prevention: Managing Environmental Factors

Plant diseases are often exacerbated by specific environmental conditions, such as high humidity or excessive leaf wetness, which can promote the growth of fungi and bacteria. Managing these environmental factors is therefore vital in preventing the outbreak and spread of diseases. Ensuring good air circulation around your plants can significantly reduce humidity levels, discouraging the development of mildew and other fungal diseases. This can be achieved by spacing plants appropriately and pruning regularly to open up the plant's structure.

Water management also plays a critical role in disease prevention. Watering plants at the soil level rather than from above reduces moisture on the leaves and stems, which can be a breeding ground for disease. If overhead watering is necessary, it should be done early in the day to allow the foliage to dry out before cooler evening temperatures set in.

Natural Remedies: Embracing Organic Solutions

When pests or diseases do occur, numerous natural remedies and organic methods can be employed before resorting to more drastic chemical treatments. Neem oil, for example, is an organic product that works against a wide variety of pests and is also effective against certain fungal diseases. It acts as an anti-feedant, repellent, and egg-laying deterrent and inhibits the development of some diseases. Garlic and chili sprays can also be homemade and used to repel pests with their strong scents.

For fungal diseases, baking soda sprays can help create an alkaline environment on the leaf surface, which is less hospitable to fungal growth. Milk is also known to be effective against powdery mildew when sprayed on affected plants. When used as part of an integrated pest and disease management strategy, these treatments can reduce the need for chemical interventions and promote a healthy, sustainable garden environment. Learn more about natural pest remedies in Appendix 7 on page 255.

Seasonal Pruning and Plant Care

Pruning Benefits: Enhancing Plant Health and Productivity Through Strategic Cuts

Pruning, the selective removal of certain parts of a plant, such as branches, buds, or roots, offers numerous benefits that significantly contribute to your garden's overall health and productivity. One of the primary advantages of regular pruning is promoting healthy growth. By removing old, dead, or diseased limbs, you allow the plant to focus its energy on developing stronger, newer growth rather than expending resources on parts that no longer benefit its overall health. This rejuvenation is particularly crucial for flowering and fruiting plants, as pruning encourages the development of new flowering buds, thereby increasing the yield of flowers and fruits.

Furthermore, pruning improves the structural integrity of plants. This practice helps shape the growth of the plants, ensuring they do not become too top-heavy or asymmetrically balanced, which could lead to physical damage during adverse weather conditions such as high winds or heavy snowfall. It also enhances the aesthetic appeal of your garden by maintaining a neat, manicured look, which can be especially important in urban settings where garden space is often visible and part of the living area.

Another significant benefit of pruning is the increased exposure to light and air among the branches. When plants become too dense, airflow is restricted, creating a humid environment conducive to developing fungal diseases. Sunlight penetration is also reduced, which can negatively affect the photosynthesis process. Strategic pruning opens the canopy to improve air circulation and light exposure, reducing disease risk and promoting a healthier plant.

Seasonal Pruning Guidelines: Timing and Techniques for Different Plants

Effective pruning is as much about when you prune as it is about how you prune. Different plants require different pruning schedules and techniques, which are often dictated by their growth cycles and seasonal changes. Spring-flowering plants, such as forsythia and azalea, typically bloom on old wood, meaning the flower buds form on branches produced in the previous year. For these plants, pruning should be done immediately after they finish blooming in late spring or early summer. This timing ensures that you do not accidentally remove the current year's flower buds, which would reduce the blooming potential for the next season.

Conversely, plants that flower in the summer, such as roses and hydrangeas, generally bloom on new wood, which means the buds form on new branches that grow in the current year. These plants are best pruned in late winter or early spring before they begin their active growth. This timing encourages vigorous new growth that will produce blooms in the same year.

For fruit trees, pruning is crucial for maintaining health and optimizing fruit size and quality. Winter pruning is common, as the trees are dormant, and the tree structure is clearly visible, allowing for more strategic cuts. However, light summer pruning can also be beneficial, especially to thin out overcrowded branches, which helps improve air circulation and sun exposure to the fruits, enhancing their ripeness and health.

The pruning technique also varies with the type of plant and your specific goals for your garden. Basic techniques include thinning, heading, and deadheading.

Thinning involves removing branches at their point of attachment to the trunk or another branch or an entire plant in densely planted areas, especially with seedlings. This method helps the plant maintain their natural shape and can increase light and air circulation for the plant and the entire garden.

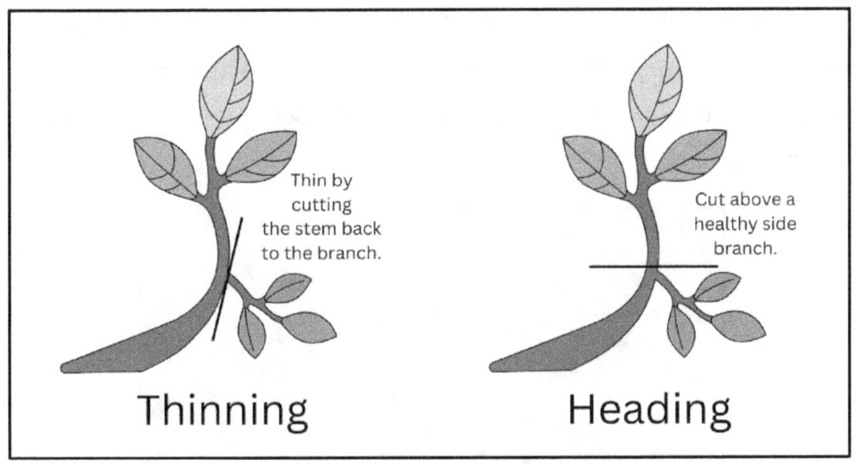

Detail of thinning vs heading cuts

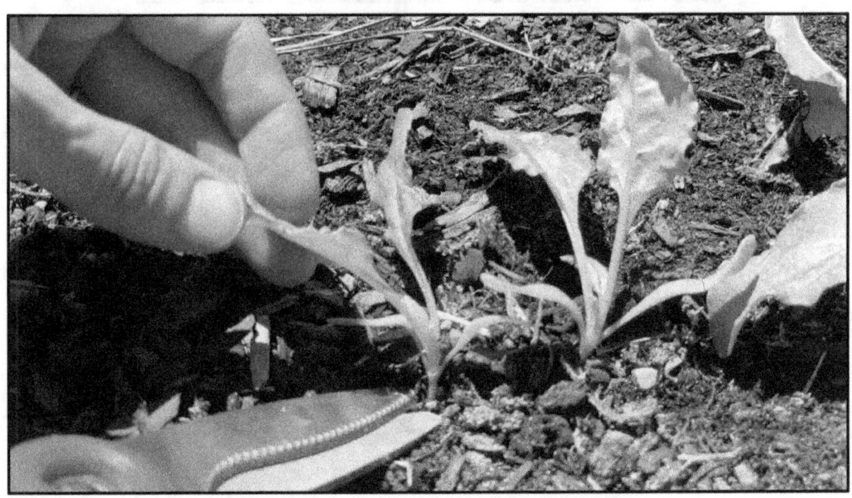

Thinning seedlings to allow for better growth

Heading involves cutting a plant back to the terminal portion of a branch to a bud. This is performed to encourage bushier growth and for shaping the plant.

Deadheading involves removing spent flowers to cleans up a plants appearance and encourage continued growth. Deadheading also directs energy into stronger growth and more flowers.

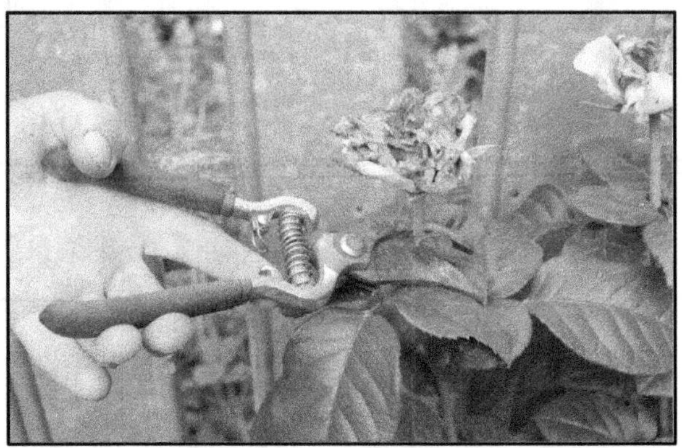

Prune below flowerhead and keep new leaves.

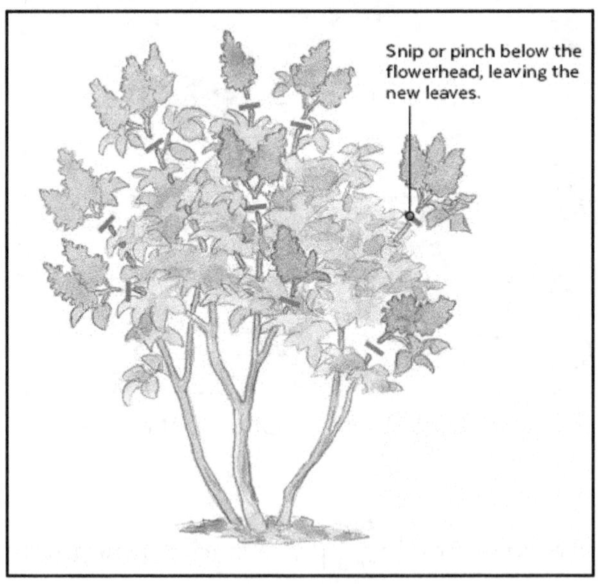

Deadheading flowers on an entire plant

Plant Support: Ensuring Stability and Growth Through Supportive Structures

As plants grow, particularly those that bear heavy fruits or flowers, providing adequate support becomes essential to prevent branches from breaking or the plant from toppling over. Supports such as stakes, trellises, or cages can ensure plants maintain their desired form and effectively manage the weight of their growth.

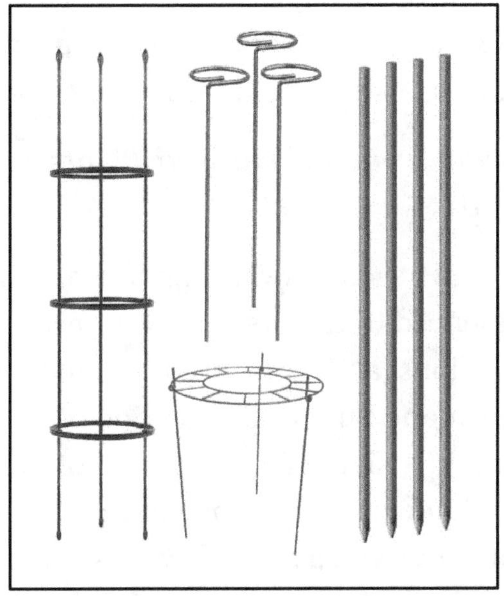

Examples of supports for plants

The type of support needed can vary widely depending on the plant species and its growth habits. Climbing plants like tomatoes or cucumbers benefit from vertical supports like cages or trellises, which allow them to grow upwards and facilitate a more productive fruiting process. For taller, non-climbing plants, such as sunflowers or delphiniums, stakes might be necessary to prevent wind damage or drooping due to the weight of their blooms.

Installing supports is best done early in the plant's growth before it becomes too large or unwieldy, as trying to add support to a fully grown plant can cause damage to the roots or the plant itself. Adjusting these supports as the plant grows is also crucial; ensure that ties and stakes are moved or loosened as needed to prevent cutting into growing stems or restricting natural growth patterns.

Seasonal Feeding: Nourishing Your Plants According to Seasonal Needs

Plant nutritional needs can vary significantly with the seasons, influenced by factors such as growth rates, weather conditions, and soil nutrient availability. As plants exit dormancy and begin a period of vigorous growth in spring, a higher concentration of nitrogen-rich fertilizers can help promote strong leaf and stem development. However, as the growing season progresses into summer, the nutritional focus should shift towards formulations that support flowering and fruiting, typically higher in phosphorus and potassium.

During the fall, reducing fertilizer application is advisable as plants prepare for dormancy; high nitrogen levels can encourage new growth that is vulnerable to winter damage. Instead, consider applying a low-nitrogen, high-potassium fertilizer to help strengthen the plants against the cold and improve root development. Over winter, most plants do not require fertilizer as their growth slows significantly; any new growth prompted by fertilization is likely to be weak and frost sensitive.

A tailored approach to feeding optimizes plant health and productivity throughout the year and contributes to the overall sustainability of your garden by ensuring that nutrients are provided efficiently and without wasteful excess.

Integrating these strategies into your gardening practice ensures that your urban garden remains a dynamic and thriving space. Seasonal pruning and plant care are not merely maintenance tasks; they are integral to your garden's ongoing success and beauty, enabling you to enjoy a lush, healthy outdoor area year-round. As we transition into the next chapter, these foundational practices will be built upon with advanced techniques that further enhance the resilience and productivity of your urban garden.

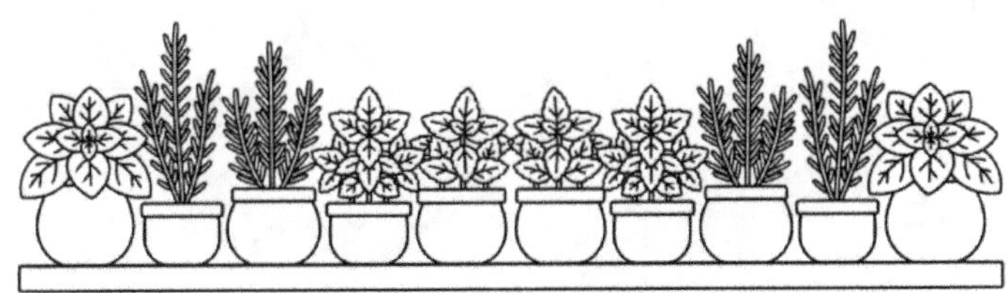

Key Chapter 4 Takeaways:

- Protect roots from cold and heat using insulation, elevation, grouping, shade cloth, and reflective surfaces, focusing on prevention before stress shows.

- Use simple monitoring tools (thermometers/sensors/weather tracking) to spot microclimate changes early and adjust plant placement in time.

- Treat light as a seasonal variable: move containers, use adjustable shade/trellises, reflect available light, and add grow lights when needed.

- Adjust watering by season: increase frequency during heat and wind, reduce in cool/damp conditions, and rely on moisture checks + mulch instead of fixed schedules.

- Reduce pest/disease pressure with strong plant care, airflow, clean-up, barriers/beneficial insects, and timely pruning/support, matched to seasonal patterns.

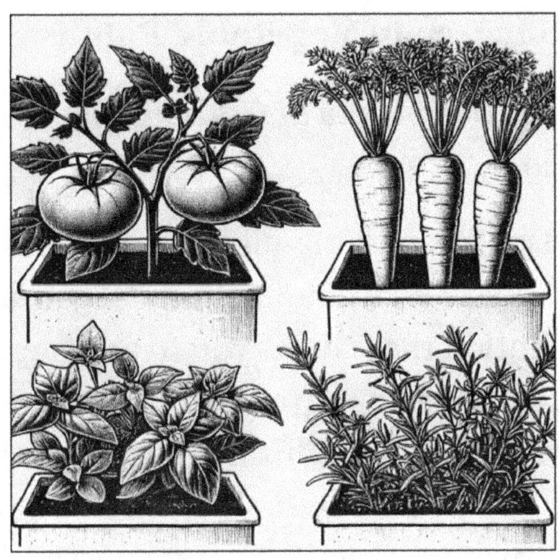

Chapter 5: Edible Gardens

Cultivating edible plants in urban environments is not just a trend but a transformative approach to integrating sustainability and self-sufficiency into daily life. For those dwelling in the heart of bustling cities, the dream of plucking fresh vegetables right from the balcony or windowsill can indeed be realized with proper guidance and an understanding of the unique challenges and opportunities urban settings present. This chapter is dedicated to helping you, the urban gardener, navigate through the process of creating a productive vegetable garden within the confines of limited space.

Starting Your Urban Vegetable Patch

Space Optimization: Vertical Gardening and Intercropping

Maximizing space is paramount in urban gardening, where every square inch counts. Vertical gardening is an innovative solution that allows you to grow upwards, effectively increasing your growing area without expanding your footprint. This method involves using trellises, wall or rail-mounted planters, and hanging baskets to cultivate a variety of vegetables, such as tomatoes, cucumbers, and beans, which naturally climb or can be easily supported to grow upward. Vertical space optimizes your limited area and adds an aesthetic dimension to your garden, creating a lush, green backdrop to your urban landscape.

Intercropping, another space-efficient strategy, involves planting different crops close together to maximize the use of space and resources. This method can be particularly effective in containers where complementary plant species are grown together; for instance, shallow-rooted herbs can be planted alongside deeper-rooted vegetables. This saves space and promotes a biodiverse environment, which can deter pests and diseases, enhancing overall garden health.

Vegetable Selection: Thriving in Containers

Choosing the right vegetables for container gardening involves considering factors such as root system size, growth habits, and environmental requirements. Vegetables like radishes, lettuce, and spinach are ideal for containers due to their compact size and short growing cycle. When planning your garden, consider the seasonality of each vegetable to ensure a continuous supply of produce. For example, cool-season crops like kale and peas can be planted in early spring or late summer, while warm-season crops like peppers and eggplants thrive when planted after the last frost.

Soil and Nutrition: Foundations of Plant Health

The vitality of your vegetable garden hinges significantly on the quality of the soil. Using a high-quality potting mix is essential in containers as it is formulated to provide proper drainage and nutrient retention. Regular fertilization is crucial to bolster plant health and productivity. Organic options such as compost, fish emulsion, or seaweed extracts feed the plants, improve soil structure, and promote beneficial microbial activity. Different vegetables have varying nutrient needs; leafy greens often require more nitrogen, while fruiting vegetables might benefit from higher phosphorus and potassium levels. Regular soil testing can provide valuable insights into nutrient levels and help tailor your fertilization practices to meet the specific needs of your garden. Learn more about nutrient solutions in Appendix 6 on page 250.

Watering Needs: Maintaining Moisture Balance

Effective watering practices are key to the success of any garden, especially in variable urban climates. Vegetables require consistent moisture to thrive, but the frequency and volume of watering will depend on factors such as plant type, growth stage, weather conditions, and the type of container used. For instance, clay pots tend to dry out faster than plastic or ceramic containers and may require more frequent watering. Employing a watering schedule that adjusts to the needs of your plants during their different growth stages ensures that they are neither overwatered nor stressed by drought, which can lead to better crop yields and reduced susceptibility to diseases.

The Benefits of Crop Rotation

Crop rotation is a powerful strategy traditionally used in large-scale agriculture that can also benefit small-scale urban gardeners. Rotating the types of vegetables grown in each container or area of your garden each season can help prevent the buildup of soil-borne pests and diseases. Additionally, different crops have varying nutrient demands; by rotating them, you can help maintain soil fertility and structure. For example, following a nitrogen-fixing legume like peas with a nitrogen-loving leafy green such as spinach can naturally replenish the soil, reducing the need for chemical fertilizers and enhancing the sustainability of your garden. This practice promotes a healthier garden and encourages you to diversify the types of vegetables you grow, increasing your culinary options and pleasure in gardening.

Herbs in Containers: Flavor at Your Fingertips

Herb gardening in urban spaces is a practical endeavor and a delightful way to infuse your daily cooking with fresh flavors directly from your balcony or windowsill. When selecting herbs for container gardening, it's paramount to choose varieties that adapt well to confined spaces and can thrive under the care of both novice and experienced gardeners. Herbs such as basil, parsley, and thyme are excellent choices due to their compact growth habits and their ability to regenerate after harvesting. These herbs provide continuous yields; for instance, basil can be picked leaf by leaf or pinched back to encourage bushier growth, ensuring a steady supply throughout the growing season. Similarly, mint spreads rapidly and can be harvested frequently, making it an ideal herb for container growing.

Harvesting techniques play a crucial role in maintaining the vitality and productivity of herb plants. Regular harvesting stimulates growth and prevents the plants from becoming woody and overgrown. It's advisable to harvest herbs early in the morning when their essential oils are at their peak, enhancing their flavors and aromas. Using sharp scissors or your fingertips, snip off what you need, always leaving enough foliage to allow the plant to continue photosynthesizing effectively. This selective and gentle harvesting method ensures your herbs remain productive and vibrant for extended periods.

The choice of containers for growing herbs is critical to their success. Herbs generally require well-draining containers to prevent water from pooling at the roots, which can lead to root rot and other fungal diseases. Materials like terracotta or clay are excellent for herb containers as they allow the soil to breathe, reducing the risk of overwatering. However, these materials can dry out quickly, especially in warmer climates, necessitating more frequent watering. The size of the container should also be considered; most herbs do well in pots at least 6-8 inches deep, which provides ample space for root development. Larger containers not only hold more soil but also retain moisture longer and are less prone to the temperature fluctuations smaller pots might experience.

Understanding the light requirements and optimal placement is crucial for plant health and flavor development when situating herb containers. Most culinary herbs, such as rosemary and oregano, thrive in full sun, requiring at least six to eight hours of direct sunlight daily. If such conditions are not feasible due to the limitations of an urban setting, herbs can still be grown successfully in partial shade, although their growth might not be as robust or their flavors as intense. Placing containers on a south-facing balcony or near a window that receives ample morning light can meet the light requirements for most herbs. For those living in particularly hot climates, providing some afternoon shade will protect herbs from scorching and help maintain moisture levels in the soil.

Watering and feeding are the final yet critical aspects of successful herb gardening in containers. Herbs prefer to be kept in slightly moist soil; overwatering can lead to several problems, including root rot and diminished flavor. Establishing a consistent watering schedule that keeps the soil lightly moist but not waterlogged is essential. During hot weather or windy days, more frequent watering may be necessary, but always check the soil moisture at a depth of about one inch to ensure watering is indeed required. In terms of nutrition, herbs do not generally require heavy fertilization. A light application of a balanced, organic fertilizer at the beginning of the growing season and perhaps once more at mid-season is sufficient. Over-fertilizing can lead to lush foliage with diluted flavor, thus defeating one of the primary joys of growing your own herbs.

By adhering to these guidelines (selecting the right herbs, using appropriate containers, placing them in optimal light conditions, and maintaining proper watering and feeding practices), you can transform even the smallest urban space into a productive and aromatic herb garden. This garden will serve as a culinary resource and a delightful green retreat that enhances your living space and cooking.

Growing Fruits in Containers: What You Need to Know

The charm of plucking fresh fruit from your garden is undeniable, and the good news for urban dwellers is that many fruit varieties can flourish right in your containers. To successfully cultivate fruit in limited spaces, understanding which varieties are most suitable for container gardening is imperative. Dwarf fruit trees and certain berry bushes are well-suited due to their compact nature and adaptability to confined environments. For instance, dwarf apple, peach, and cherry tree varieties have been specifically bred to have smaller root systems and mature sizes, making them ideal for container life. These trees can provide delicious fruits and add a delightful aesthetic element to your urban space. Similarly, berry plants such as strawberries, blueberries, and raspberries can thrive in containers, offering bountiful harvests if their specific soil and sun exposure needs are met.

In addition to selecting the right varieties, understanding the pollination requirements of your fruit plants is crucial for ensuring successful fruit production. Many fruit trees, including apples and pears, are not self-pollinating and require pollen from another tree of a different variety to produce fruit. In the constrained spaces of an urban garden, planting two compatible varieties might not always be feasible. In such cases, opting for self-pollinating varieties, or those that require only one plant to produce fruit, such as certain types of peaches and citrus fruits, can be a practical solution. For urban settings where attracting natural pollinators might be challenging, manual pollination can also be effective by gently transferring pollen from one flower to another with a small brush. Ensuring your plants are accessible to pollinators by placing them in areas free from high winds and heavy pollution can further enhance pollination success.

Potting and repotting play pivotal roles in the health and productivity of container-grown fruit plants. Choosing the correct pot size is essential from the start; a pot that is too small can restrict root growth and limit the plant's development, while an overly large pot can lead to waterlogging issues, which might harm the roots. Generally, a pot allowing about 2 to 3 inches of extra space around the root ball is ideal for initial planting. As the plant grows, repotting may be necessary to accommodate the expanding root system. This is typically done every few years before the roots become too crowded, which can lead to decreased fruit yields. When repotting, it's also an excellent opportunity to refresh the soil, which can become depleted of nutrients over time. Using a high-quality potting mix designed for the specific type of fruit plant you are growing will provide the best results.

Pruning and ongoing care are integral to maintaining a healthy and productive fruit garden in containers. Regular pruning helps shape the plant, control its size, and encourage new fruiting wood growth. For most fruit trees, the best time to prune is during the dormant season (late winter or early spring) before new growth begins. This timing lets you easily see the tree's structure and make precise cuts. The goal of pruning should be to remove any dead or diseased branches, thin out over-crowded areas to improve air circulation, and cut back overly vigorous branches that can sap energy from the developing fruits. Additionally, seasonal care should include monitoring for pests and diseases, which can be more prevalent in container plants due to the restricted growing conditions. Implementing regular inspections and treating with appropriate organic pesticides or fungicides when issues are detected can help keep your plants healthy.

You can transform your urban space into a fruitful oasis by understanding these key aspects: selecting suitable fruit varieties, managing pollination, potting and repotting appropriately, and maintaining rigorous pruning and care routines. These efforts enhance the sustainability of your gardening practice and bring the joy of fresh, home-grown fruits to your table, making urban gardening a truly rewarding endeavor.

Companion Planting for Container Edibles

Companion planting represents a venerable practice deeply rooted in agricultural wisdom, offering multiple benefits that are particularly significant in the confined spaces of urban container gardens. Learn more about plants that grow well together in Appendix 2 on page 236. This method involves placing plants in proximity that mutually benefit from each other through pest control, nutrient uptake, or growth enhancement. The essence of companion planting is in creating a harmonious community of plants where each species contributes to the health and productivity of its neighbors. This symbiotic planting strategy not only optimizes the use of limited space but also fosters a balanced ecosystem that can naturally deter pests and enhance plant growth.

One of the fundamental advantages of companion planting is the natural pest control it offers. Certain plants emit fragrances or chemicals that can repel harmful insects, thereby protecting more vulnerable plant species. For example, marigolds are well-known for their ability to deter nematodes and other pests through a substance they release into the soil, which makes them excellent companions for tomatoes and peppers. Similarly, the strong scent of herbs like basil and mint can confuse pests looking for their favorite host plants, such as tomatoes and cabbage, respectively. By strategically placing these plants alongside susceptible varieties, you can reduce the need for chemical pesticides, leading to a healthier, more sustainable garden environment.

Moreover, companion planting can enhance the growth and health of your plants. Legumes, such as beans and peas, have the ability to fix atmospheric nitrogen into the soil, enriching it for nitrogen-loving plants like spinach and lettuce. When these plants are grown together in the same container or adjacent containers, the legumes supply the extra nitrogen their companions need, promoting lush, vigorous growth. This natural method of nutrient sharing improves soil fertility and reduces the need for synthetic fertilizers, which can be especially beneficial in the limited soil volumes of container gardens.

When implementing companion planting in containers, understanding ideal plant combinations is crucial. Plants with similar water and light needs but different root depths can be paired effectively in the same container. For example, shallow-rooted herbs like cilantro or chives can be planted with deeper-rooted vegetables like carrots or beets. This arrangement allows both types of plants to thrive without competing for the same soil resources. Additionally, tall sun-loving plants, such as tomatoes, can be paired with low-growing, shade-tolerant plants, such as lettuce, which can benefit from the shade provided by the taller plants during hot weather.

Spacing and Layout: Maximizing Mutual Benefits

Effective spacing and layout are vital in companion planting to ensure that each plant has sufficient space to grow without hindrance. In containers, it is particularly important to consider the mature size of each plant and arrange them so that they have enough room to reach their full potential. Plants placed too closely can compete for light, water, and nutrients, stunting growth and making them more susceptible to diseases and pests. To avoid this, always adhere to the spacing guidelines suggested for each plant variety, adjusting as necessary for their combined growth in a shared container.

A staggered or tiered arrangement can be beneficial in containers, allowing each plant access to adequate sunlight and air circulation. For instance, taller plants can be placed at the back of a rectangular container, with shorter plants in the front, ensuring that all plants receive sunlight. Alternatively, a tiered planter can help achieve the same effect in a vertical space, making it ideal for balconies or small patios.

Avoiding Competition: Navigating Plant Relationships

While many plants benefit from being grown together, some combinations should be avoided due to their antagonistic relationships Learn more about what plants do not grow well together in Appendix 3 on page 240. Some plants can be overly competitive, stunting the growth of their neighbors by aggressively depleting shared resources or secreting substances that inhibit other plants' growth. For example, planting garlic or onions near beans or peas can inhibit the growth of legumes, as alliums can interfere with the growth of leguminous plants. Similarly, fennel is a poor companion for most garden plants because it secretes substances that inhibit growth in many other plants.

Understanding these relationships is crucial in planning your container garden to ensure that plant interactions are beneficial rather than detrimental. Consulting companion planting charts can guide which plants are compatible and which are not. By carefully selecting and positioning your plants, you can create a cooperative community of container edibles that survive and thrive, providing a bountiful and beautiful harvest.

Pollinator-Friendly Gardening in Small Spaces

Pollinators play a pivotal role in the health of our planet's ecosystems, facilitating the reproduction of many plants by transferring pollen from one flower to another. This leads to fruit and seed production and promotes genetic diversity in the plant population. In urban environments, where natural habitats are often scarce, creating pollinator-friendly spaces can significantly impact the local biodiversity. By attracting pollinators such as bees, butterflies, and hummingbirds to your garden, you contribute to the conservation of these essential species while also enhancing the productivity and health of your plants. Pollinators are particularly crucial for the fruiting process in many plants; without their diligent pollination work, yields could be drastically reduced, and the quality of fruits and vegetables would likely decline.

Attracting pollinators to an urban garden requires thoughtful planning and specific practices. Learn more about pollinator plant options in Appendix 4 on page 244. The first step is the selection of plants known to attract these beneficial creatures. Varieties such as lavender, salvia, and marigold are renowned for attracting bees, while butterfly bushes and milkweed are favorites among butterflies. Including a range of plants that flower at different times of the year ensures that pollinators have a consistent source of nectar and pollen, crucial for their survival and continual presence in your garden. These plants serve pollinators' needs and add vibrant colors and fragrances to your space, enhancing its aesthetic appeal.

In addition to plant selection, creating a welcoming habitat for pollinators involves providing them with the necessities of survival: food, water, and shelter. Small water features such as a birdbath or even shallow dishes of water can offer vital hydration to these visitors. Be sure to include stones or floating pieces of wood to provide safe landing spots to prevent drowning. Shelter can be provided in the form of natural foliage or artificial bug hotels, which offer refuge for various pollinators. These simple additions can make your garden a haven for pollinators, encouraging them to return and assisting in pollinating your plants throughout the season.

The use of pesticides, even those labeled as organic or natural, can be detrimental to pollinators. Thus, adopting integrated pest management (IPM) practices that focus on prevention, monitoring, and controlling pests through natural means is crucial. Techniques such as encouraging beneficial insects that prey on harmful pests, using barriers to protect plants, and manually removing pests can effectively manage garden health without resorting to harmful chemicals. When interventions are necessary, opting for targeted and targeted treatments during times when pollinators are least active, such as at dusk, can mitigate potential harm to these vital creatures.

By integrating these practices into your gardening routine, you enhance the ecological value of your urban space and contribute to the broader environmental efforts to support pollinator populations. This holistic approach to gardening encourages a symbiotic relationship with nature, fostering a balanced ecosystem where both plants and pollinators thrive, enhancing the beauty and productivity of your garden.

In conclusion, this chapter underscores the importance of creating pollinator-friendly environments within urban settings. By choosing the right plants, providing essential resources, and avoiding harmful chemicals, you can turn your garden into a sanctuary for beneficial pollinators.

This contributes to global biodiversity efforts and enriches your gardening experience by ensuring a flourishing, productive garden. As we move forward, these principles of sustainability and environmental stewardship will continue to guide our gardening practices, ensuring that our green spaces serve our needs and those of the natural world around us.

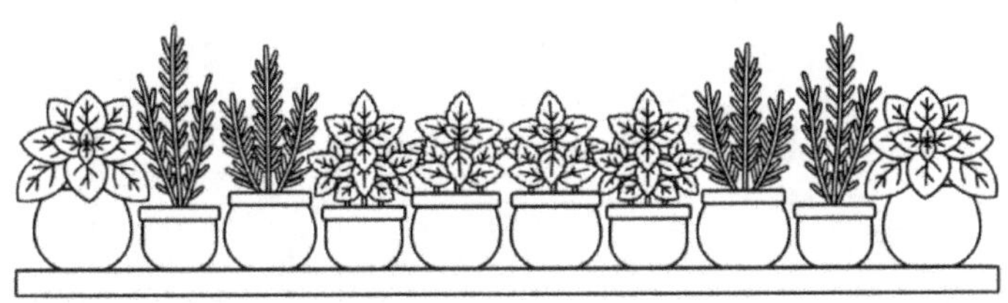

Key Chapter 5 Takeaways:

- Maximize harvest in limited space with vertical supports, rail/wall planters, hanging containers, and intercropping that pairs compatible plants.

- Choose container-friendly edibles based on root depth, growth habit, and season timing so your planting plan stays realistic and productive.

- Prioritize strong foundations: high-quality potting mix, regular feeding, and moisture consistency (especially in containers that dry quickly).

- Grow herbs and fruits successfully by matching container size, drainage, sunlight, pruning needs, and pollination requirements to the plant.

- Increase yields naturally by using companion planting + pollinator-friendly plants + low-chemical IPM practices to support a balanced mini-ecosystem.

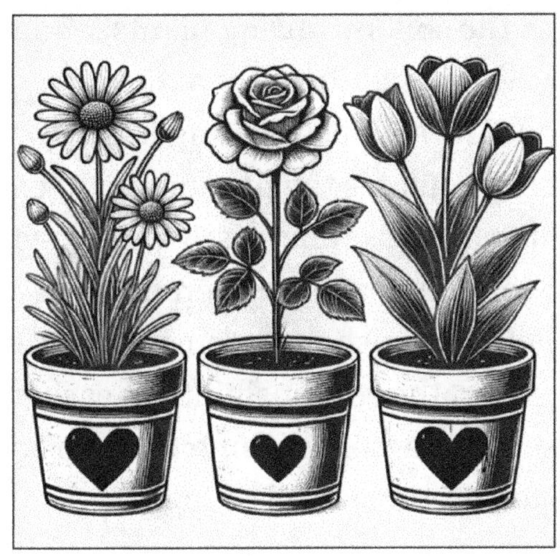

Chapter 6: Decorative and Therapeutic Gardening

Amid the hustle and bustle of urban life, finding a tranquil retreat can significantly enhance one's quality of life. Gardening, often perceived purely as a means to beautify or produce food, holds profound therapeutic qualities that can transform spaces and the mental and emotional well-being of those who engage in it. This chapter delves into the lesser-discussed aspect of gardening and its role as a powerful form of stress relief and a conduit for mindfulness and personal reflection.

Gardening as a Form of Stress Relief

Gardening offers a unique therapeutic benefit, providing a peaceful escape from the pressures of daily urban living.

Engaging with the soil, nurturing plants, and witnessing the growth cycle can significantly reduce stress and improve mood. The act of gardening involves physical activity, which stimulates the production of endorphins, the body's natural stress relievers. This physical engagement, combined with the serene environment of a garden, can help diminish symptoms of depression and anxiety. Moreover, the responsibility of caring for plants can instill a sense of accomplishment and pride, further contributing to emotional well-being.

Incorporating mindfulness techniques into gardening practices can enhance these therapeutic benefits. Mindful gardening involves being fully present in the gardening activity by focusing on the senses, like feeling the texture of the soil, hearing the rustle of leaves, seeing the vibrant colors of the flowers, and smelling the earthiness of the ground. This practice helps anchor the gardener in the present moment, cultivating a state of mindfulness that has been shown to reduce stress and promote mental clarity.

To deepen this experience, consider growing sensory plants in your garden. Sensory plants are varieties known for their soothing scents, interesting textures, or visually calming colors. Lavender, with its soft fragrance, is renowned for reducing stress and encouraging relaxation. Chamomile, another plant known for its calming properties, can be easily grown and used to make herbal tea, providing a soothing ritual to end a gardening session. Incorporating these plants enhances the garden's aesthetic and increases its role as a therapeutic space.

Transforming your gardening space into a personal retreat involves more than just plant selection; it requires thoughtful consideration of the overall environment. Creating secluded nooks within the garden using trellises covered with climbing plants or arranging the garden furniture to face away from the distractions of the outside world can help establish a more intimate and peaceful setting. Adding elements such as soft, flowing fabrics or gentle wind chimes can enhance the sensory experience, making the garden a perfect place for relaxation and reflection.

Interactive Element: Mindful Gardening Exercise

To help you integrate mindfulness into your gardening routine, consider this simple exercise: Next time you are in your garden, take a moment to close your eyes and take three deep breaths, focusing solely on the sounds around you. Try being aware of the chirping of birds, the rustling of leaves, or the distant hum of city life. Open your eyes and spend a few minutes observing the details of a single plant, noting the patterns of its leaves, the texture of its stem, and the shades of its colors. This practice of attentive observation can help center your mind, reduce feelings of stress, and increase your appreciation of the natural beauty in your care.

Flowers and Foliage: Making Your Space Bloom

Adding flowers and foliage to your urban garden transforms mere living spaces into vibrant sanctuaries bursting with color and life. When selecting plants for such environments, it is paramount to choose varieties that thrive in confined spaces and contribute significantly to your garden's visual appeal. Compact growth habits and significant ornamental value are key traits to look for. Flowers such as petunias and marigolds are excellent choices due to their bright, long-lasting blooms and relatively small root systems, making them ideal for container cultivation. For foliage, consider ferns and hostas, which offer lush greenery and texture to garden compositions without requiring extensive horizontal space.

In applying design principles to your garden, using color theory and texture plays a crucial role in creating visually appealing arrangements. Color theory in garden design involves understanding the relationships between colors on the color wheel to create harmonious combinations. For example, complementary colors, such as blue and orange, can enhance your garden display's visual impact. Similarly, incorporating a variety of textures can add depth and interest. The soft fronds of ferns juxtaposed with the glossy leaves of hostas provide a tactile diversity that invites interest and interaction. These principles are not merely aesthetic considerations but are strategic in making small spaces appear larger and more inviting.

Seasonal blooms are essential for maintaining year-round vibrancy in your garden. Integrating a mix of perennials and annuals ensures a continuous display of color. Perennials such as daylilies and sedums offer longevity and return each year with minimal maintenance, providing a reliable backbone for your garden's aesthetic. Supplement these with annuals like impatiens and snapdragons, which can fill in gaps and offer bright pops of color throughout the growing season. Considering their blooming cycles, the strategic layering of these plants ensures that as one plant's flowers begin to fade, another's just beginning to flourish, maintaining an ever-evolving display.

Maintaining these floral displays requires attention to garden care practices that extend the life and beauty of your plants. Regular deadheading of spent flowers is aesthetically necessary and promotes further blooming by preventing plants from going to seed. This technique encourages plants to focus energy back into flower production rather than seed development. Dividing perennials every few years is another important maintenance task that prevents container overcrowding and rejuvenates the plant by giving it more room to grow and access nutrients. This process involves removing the plant from its container, cutting it into smaller sections, and replanting these divisions in the same container with fresh soil or new containers. This revitalizes your existing plants and can help expand your garden without additional cost.

By integrating these thoughtful selections and maintenance practices, your urban gardening efforts can yield a flourishing oasis that offers a visual feast and a dynamic, ever-changing tapestry of nature's best displays.

Creating a Zen Garden in a Container

The concept of a Zen Garden, originating from traditional Japanese garden design, focuses on achieving a meditative and tranquil environment through simplicity and natural beauty. These gardens are characterized by their minimalist approach, incorporating elements such as rocks, sand, and carefully selected plants to create a serene and contemplative space. When adapting this concept to container gardening, particularly in urban settings where space and peace are at a premium, the same principles apply but on a smaller scale.

Key elements of a Zen Garden include rocks and sand, which symbolize the natural landscape. Rocks can represent mountains, while sand suggests water, raked into patterns that mimic the ripple of waves. In a container setting, selecting the right size and color of rocks becomes crucial; they should be proportionate to the size of the container and harmoniously colored to evoke a naturalistic feel. Sand, or fine gravel, should be clean and light in color, offering a contrast that highlights the rocks, and any plants used. Raking the sand in various patterns serves aesthetic purposes and becomes a mindful activity, helping to center thoughts and focus the mind.

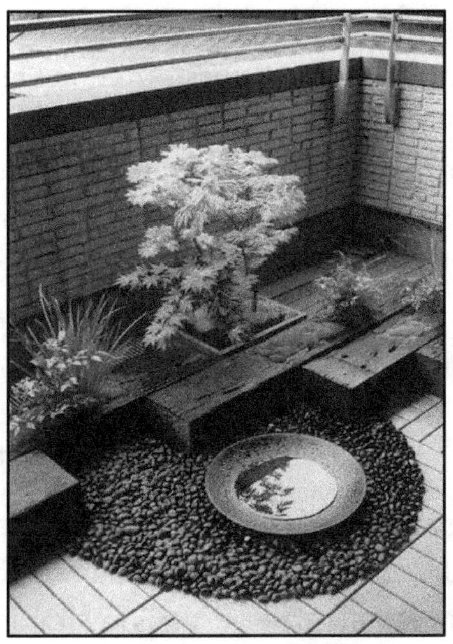

Example of a Zen Garden

When choosing a container for your Zen Garden, simplicity and tranquility are the guiding principles. Containers in neutral colors such as blacks, grays, or earth tones are ideal as they do not distract from the elements within. The shape of the container should be simple and elegant, avoiding any ornate designs that might disrupt the minimalist aesthetic essential to Zen philosophy. Materials such as stone, ceramic, or high-quality resin that mimic natural textures are preferable. The container's depth must accommodate the elements you wish to include, such as rocks, which may need a substantial base for stability and enough sand to allow for raking.

Arranging the elements within your Zen Garden requires a thoughtful approach to maintain balance and harmony. Start by placing larger rocks first, thinking about how they relate to each other and the container's edges. These rocks should be placed deliberately, often in odd numbers, and with consideration to their best angles. Once the rocks are positioned, add the sand, ensuring it is evenly spread before beginning the meditative practice of raking. Patterns in the sand should flow and change, representing water around the rocks, and can be adjusted according to your mood or the desired focus of your meditation.

Incorporating a water feature into your container Zen Garden introduces an additional element of calmness and movement. For small-scale gardens, a simple bamboo waterspout or a small recirculating fountain can add the soothing sound of trickling water, enhancing the sensory experience of the garden. The water feature should not overwhelm the garden's simplicity but rather complement the other elements, maintaining the minimalist aesthetic. Placement should consider practical aspects such as access to water and electricity for pumps and visual balance within the container.

Creating a Zen Garden in a container offers a unique opportunity to bring traditional Zen gardens' calming and meditative qualities into the compact spaces typical of urban environments. By carefully selecting and arranging elements such as rocks, sand, and water features within a suitably simple container, you can establish a personal sanctuary that provides aesthetic pleasure and a peaceful retreat from the stresses of urban life. This miniature landscape becomes a tool for personal reflection and tranquility, an ever-present invitation to pause and immerse in the moment, fostering a deeper connection with the natural world.

Attracting Wildlife to Your Urban Garden

Fostering a connection between urban environments and wildlife can transform even the smallest garden into a vibrant habitat, contributing positively to local biodiversity and offering a unique opportunity to observe nature's interplay at close quarters. Selecting the right plants is crucial when cultivating a garden that invites birds, butterflies, and beneficial insects. These should thrive in confined spaces and provide the necessary resources (nectar, pollen, and seeds) to attract and sustain wildlife.

For instance, consider incorporating native plant species, which are often more attractive to local wildlife due to their co-evolutionary relationships. Plants like Echinacea (coneflower) and Rudbeckia (black-eyed Susan) are excellent for attracting butterflies and bees due to their ample nectar. Additionally, their seeds can provide food for birds during the autumn months. Similarly, Lavandula (lavender) can be a magnet for bees, while its dense foliage offers shelter to beneficial insects. Planting a variety of these species ensures that your garden blooms with life throughout the growing season and supports a range of wildlife, each attracted by specific plant characteristics.

Including water sources in your urban garden greatly enhances its appeal to wildlife, providing a vital resource that attracts birds, insects, and even small mammals. This can be achieved in small spaces through compact features such as bird baths or small, self-contained water fountains, which can be placed on balconies or patios. It is essential to keep these water sources clean and replenish them regularly to prevent the spread of diseases. Adding a few stones or pebbles to the water features can provide safe landing spots for insects and small birds, preventing drowning while allowing them to drink safely.

Providing shelter and nesting materials is another fundamental aspect of creating a wildlife-friendly garden. This can be as simple as leaving some of your garden a little wild, with piles of leaves or twigs that can offer nesting materials and hiding spots for small creatures. Installing birdhouses or insect hotels can be an effective alternative for those who prefer a tidier space. These structures should be placed in quiet, sheltered parts of the garden to offer safe refuge from predators and harsh weather. Ensuring these shelters are made from natural, untreated materials is key to avoiding substances that could be harmful to wildlife.

Balancing the needs of wildlife with the enjoyment of human occupants requires thoughtful garden planning and management. To ensure that your garden remains a pleasant space for both people and animals, it is important to position wildlife-friendly plants and features so that they can be easily observed from your living areas or while you are tending to the garden. This allows for the enjoyment of watching wildlife and makes it easier to manage and maintain the garden without causing disturbance. Regular monitoring and maintenance of the garden, such as controlling the growth of plants and cleaning water features, ensure that it remains attractive and functional for human use while still providing the necessary resources for wildlife.

By integrating into your urban garden the elements of wildlife-friendly plants, water sources, shelters, and a thoughtful layout, it can become a sanctuary for you and local wildlife. This not only enhances the ecological value of urban spaces but also enriches your gardening experience, offering daily encounters with the natural world right at your doorstep. As we continue to explore the multifaceted benefits of urban gardening, these practices underline the potential of small spaces to contribute significantly to urban biodiversity and the well-being of its human and wildlife inhabitants.

Night Gardens: Plants That Shine After Sunset

The enchantment of a garden need not fade with the setting sun. Night gardens, designed to peak after dusk, offer a unique allure with blooms that glow under the moonlight and fragrances that waft through the evening air. This garden type enhances the sensory experience of your outdoor space and extends its usability, allowing you to enjoy its tranquility during the cooler, quieter hours. Plants that bloom or release their fragrance at night can transform a simple balcony or patio into an enchanting nocturnal retreat.

Night-blooming plants such as Moonflower, Evening Primrose, and Night Phlox are perfect for these settings. With its large, white blooms, Moonflower opens only at night, filling the air with a sweet fragrance, while Evening Primrose's yellow flowers add a subtle glow and a fresh scent. These plants do more than just beautify; they create a dynamic environment that evolves from day to night, offering new textures and aromas that are absent during daylight hours. This transformation adds a layer of intrigue and mystery to your garden, making each evening a new discovery.

To enhance the visual appeal of your night garden, consider integrating garden-friendly lighting that accentuates the beauty of nocturnal blooms without overwhelming them. Soft, ambient lighting can be achieved by strategically placing solar-powered lights that mimic the natural glow of moonlight. Position these lights beneath plants to illuminate their foliage and flowers, casting dramatic shadows and highlighting their forms against the dark sky. Alternatively, installing low-voltage LED lights along pathways or around seating areas can provide gentle illumination that enhances safety and creates a welcoming atmosphere, encouraging relaxation and contemplation during the evening hours.

Designing your garden for evening enjoyment involves more than just choosing the right plants and lights. It requires thoughtful consideration of how the space will be used at night. Seating should be comfortable and arranged to encourage relaxation or social interaction. Consider adding elements that appeal to the senses, such as a small fountain whose gentle sound complements the quiet of the evening or a fire pit that provides warmth and a central gathering spot. These elements can make your night garden a visual delight and a functional extension of your living space.

Attracting nocturnal wildlife can further enrich the ecosystem of your night garden. Many pollinators, such as certain moths and bats, are active at night and are attracted to white or pale-colored flowers that are visible under low-light conditions. Planting a variety of these can support local biodiversity and contribute to the health of your garden. Additionally, including features such as a small water dish or bird bath can provide essential resources for nocturnal wildlife, encouraging them to visit your garden and assist in pollination.

Integrating these elements (night-blooming plants, subtle lighting, thoughtful design, and wildlife-friendly features) creates a garden that captivates the senses and serves as a peaceful refuge at the end of the day. This chapter has explored the unique aspects of night gardening, from selecting plants that thrive in the cooler, darker hours to creating a space that invites both human and animal visitors to enjoy its nocturnal offerings. As we transition from the magic of night gardens, the next chapter will delve into innovative gardening methods that further harness modern technologies and practices to enhance the urban gardening experience. This exploration will provide the tools and knowledge to expand your gardening capabilities, embracing new techniques that can revolutionize how you interact with your urban environment.

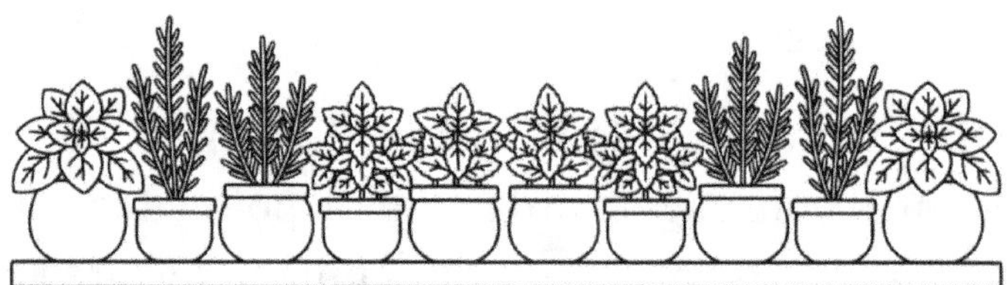

Key Chapter 6 Takeaways:

- Use gardening as a reset: focus on simple, sensory moments (touch, scent, sound, color) to support calm and reduce stress.

- Choose plants with sensory value (fragrance, texture, soothing color) to make your space feel like a personal retreat, not just a project.

- Build visual impact in small spaces with compact blooms, foliage contrast, seasonal layering, and routine care like deadheading and dividing.

- Create a container Zen garden by keeping elements simple and intentional (rocks, sand/gravel, balanced placement, optional small water feature).

- Support biodiversity by adding native or wildlife-friendly plants, clean water sources, and shelter, and consider a night garden with pale blooms and gentle lighting for evening enjoyment.

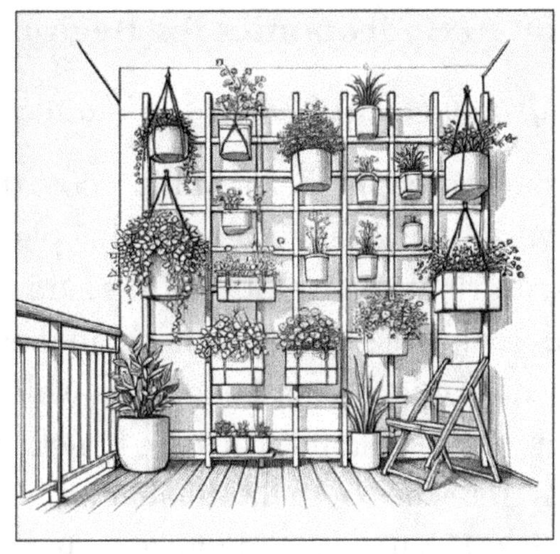

Chapter 7: Innovative Gardening Methods

In the realm of urban gardening, space constraints and the quest for efficiency drive the need for innovative approaches that maximize productivity and ease of maintenance. One such method, revolutionizing the way city dwellers cultivate plants, is hydroponics. This technique, which might sound intricate at first, is actually quite accessible and offers a plethora of benefits to the urban gardener. Hydroponics, the art of growing plants without soil, uses nutrient-rich water solutions to nurture plants, resulting in higher yields and rapid growth. This method conserves space and water and eliminates many common garden pests and diseases associated with soil cultivation.

Introduction to Hydroponics for Beginners

Basics of Hydroponics: Cultivating Without Soil

Hydroponics may seem modern, but its roots trace back to ancient civilizations. It involves growing plants in a water-based, nutrient-rich solution, thus skipping the need for soil. Roots are supported using an inert medium such as perlite, vermiculite, or peat moss, which helps physically support the plants. The core benefit of hydroponic systems lies in their efficiency and control. Nutrient levels, pH balance, and moisture in the growing environment can be precisely controlled, allowing plants to receive exactly what they need for optimal growth. This control maximizes plant health and yield and allows for faster growth compared to traditional soil-based gardening. For urban gardeners with limited space, hydroponics offers a compact, soil-free solution for growing everything from herbs to vegetables.

Setting Up a Simple System: A Beginner's Guide

For those new to hydroponics, starting simple is key. A basic hydroponic setup suitable for beginners is the wick system. This passive system requires no pumps or electricity, making it ideal for those just starting out. You will need an air-tight container, a growing medium, wick, nutrient solution, and your plants. The wick system draws nutrient-rich solution from a reservoir into the growing medium via capillary action, which feeds the plants. It's an excellent method for growing smaller, less water-intensive plants like herbs and lettuce. As you gain confidence, you may explore more complex systems such as the deep-water culture (DWC) or the nutrient film technique (NFT), which allow for greater yield and plant variety.

Nutrient Solutions: The Lifeline of Hydroponics

The heartbeat of any hydroponic system is its nutrient solution. This liquid replaces all the benefits of soil, supplying plants with the essential minerals and nutrients required for growth. Creating the right nutrient mix involves understanding the specific needs of your plants at different stages of their growth. Most hydroponic shops offer pre-mixed solutions or concentrated nutrients you can dilute with water. For those who prefer a more hands-on approach, mixing your solutions from individual elements can be more economical and allows customized nutrient blends. Regularly monitor the electrical conductivity (EC) with a simple meter to ensure nutrient levels remain optimal for your plants' current growth stages.

Maintenance and Monitoring: Ensuring System Health

Maintaining a hydroponic system involves regular monitoring and cleaning to ensure optimal operation and plant health. pH levels should be checked weekly, as the absorption of different nutrients is pH dependent. Ideally, keep the pH between 5.5 and 6.5, adjusting the pH up or down solutions as needed. System cleaning should be performed every few weeks to prevent the buildup of salts and other residues, which can clog the system and harm your plants. This involves flushing the system with clean water and replacing the nutrient solution entirely to ensure a fresh environment for your plants to thrive.

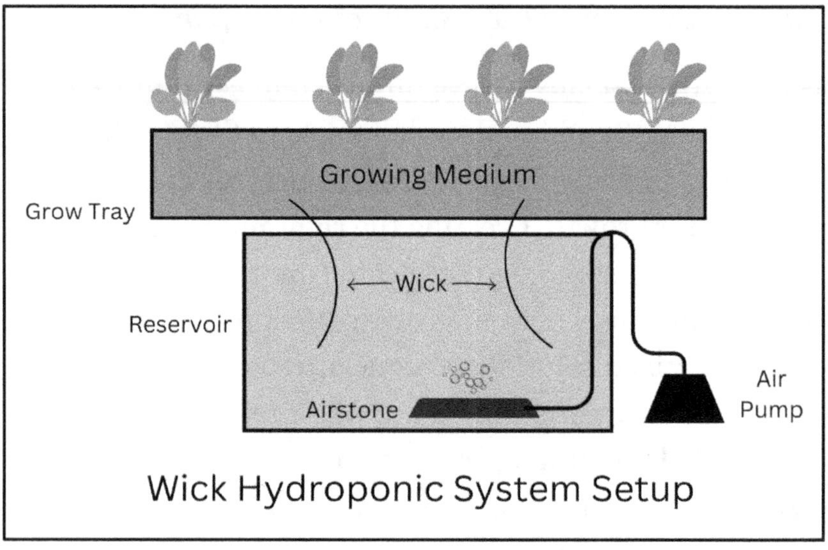

Detail of a hydroponic garden system setup

In embracing hydroponics, you are not only adopting a method that saves space and water but also engaging with a form of gardening that offers precise control over the growing environment, leading to healthier plants and more abundant yields. This chapter serves as your introduction to the world of soil-less gardening, a technique that fits perfectly with the urban lifestyle, where efficiency and productivity are paramount. As you explore further, each step forward in this hydroponic adventure opens up new possibilities for cultivating a thriving garden in the city's heart.

Exploring Aquaponics in Urban Gardening

Aquaponics, a system that combines aquaculture (raising fish) and hydroponics (soil-less plant cultivation), offers an intriguing solution for urban gardeners. This symbiotic environment, where fish and plants thrive together, epitomizes sustainability and efficiency. In aquaponics, fish waste provides an organic nutrient source for the plants, while the plants naturally filter and purify the water, which is then recirculated back to the fish. This closed-loop system reduces the need for chemical fertilizers and conserves water, making it an ideal choice for eco-conscious urban dwellers seeking to maximize limited gardening spaces.

For those new to aquaponics, understanding the basic setup involves a few key components: a fish tank, a grow bed where plants are held, a water pump, and a filtration system to manage waste. The beauty of aquaponics lies in its scalability, making it suitable for small balconies or larger gardens. Starting with a small-scale system can be as simple as using a standard aquarium for fish, paired with a grow bed above it supported by a sturdy frame. Water is pumped from the fish tank to the grow bed, where it percolates through the growing medium, delivering nutrients to the plant roots before being filtered and returned to the tank.

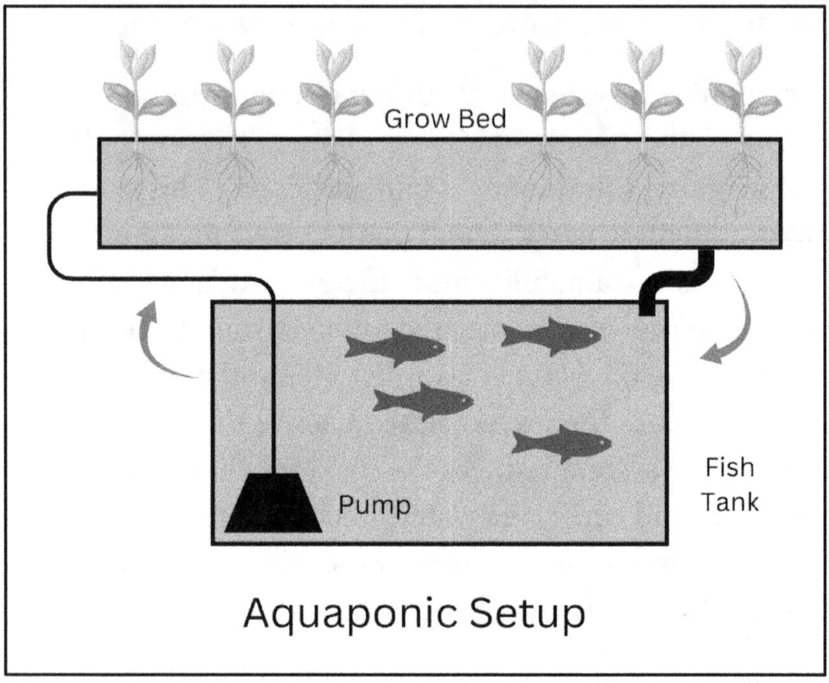

Detail of an aquaponic garden setup

The right fish and plants are crucial for maintaining a balanced aquaponic system. Fish commonly used include tilapia and goldfish due to their hardiness and adaptability to different environmental conditions. However, the choice of fish might be influenced by local regulations, personal preferences, and the size of the setup, including whether the fish are intended for consumption. When it comes to plants, species that thrive on high-nutrient uptake, such as leafy greens and herbs, are particularly well-suited for aquaponics. Learn more about suitable hydroponic plants in Appendix 5 on page 246. These include lettuce, basil, and watercress. The key is to avoid plants that require acidic conditions, as most aquaponic systems tend to run slightly alkaline. Learn more about plants to avoid while hydroponic gardening in Appendix 5 on page 249.

Maintaining an aquaponic system requires attention to water quality and system balance. Regularly monitoring pH levels, ammonia, nitrite, and nitrate concentrations is essential to ensure a healthy environment for fish and plants. The pH should ideally be maintained around 6.8 to 7.0, which is generally acceptable for most plants and fish. Ammonia levels must be closely monitored, especially in new systems, as high levels can be toxic to fish. This involves routine testing and adjustments to the feeding rates or plant densities to manage nutrient levels effectively.

Incorporating aquaponics into urban gardening initiatives not only optimizes the use of limited space but also contributes to sustainable living practices. By fostering a system where water is recycled, and chemical inputs are minimized, urban gardeners can enjoy the dual benefits of home-grown produce and fresh fish, all from the convenience of their balcony or rooftop. As urban agriculture continues to evolve, aquaponics stands out as a particularly innovative and beneficial method, blending simplicity with ecological responsibility.

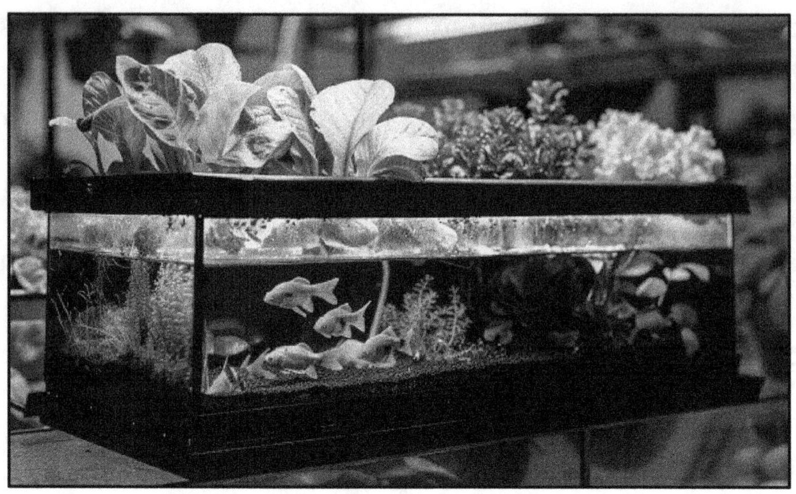

Example of a mature aquaponic garden setup

Smart Gardening: Leveraging Technology

Technology plays a pivotal role in the modern urban garden, seamlessly integrating into daily gardening routines to enhance efficiency, precision, and productivity. As we delve into the realm of smart gardening, we uncover an array of technological tools designed to simplify the complexities of garden management. These innovations are not merely gadgets; they are transformative tools that cater to urban gardeners' unique needs, making gardening more accessible and less time-consuming.

Technological Tools for Gardening: Enhancing Precision and Ease

Technology integration into gardening begins with tools that assist in basic but crucial tasks. Soil moisture sensors, for instance, are invaluable in providing real-time data on the water content of the soil, eliminating the guesswork in watering schedules. These sensors can be particularly beneficial in container gardening, where maintaining optimal moisture levels is critical due to the limited soil volume. Similarly, plant identification apps have revolutionized how gardeners understand their plants. By simply taking a photograph, these apps can identify species, diagnose plant diseases, and offer care instructions, which is especially helpful for beginners unfamiliar with the vast variety of plants suitable for urban environments.

Automating Garden Care: Streamlining Routine Tasks

Automating daily gardening tasks saves time and ensures that plants receive consistent care. Self-watering containers exemplify this automation, equipped with reservoirs that allow plants to absorb water as needed through capillary action. This system effectively prevents overwatering and underwatering, common issues in manually managed urban gardens. Additionally, smart irrigation systems can be programmed to water plants based on specific schedules or in response to soil moisture data collected by sensors. These systems can adjust water flow based on weather conditions by reducing water use on rainy days and increasing it during dry spells thereby enhancing water conservation while ensuring plants remain hydrated.

Adopting automated nutrient delivery systems further simplifies the process of fertilizing plants. These systems can dispense the right amount of nutrients at designated times, reducing waste and ensuring optimal plant growth. By integrating with sensors that monitor nutrient levels in the soil, these systems can adjust their outputs, applying more precise fertilizer amounts tailored to the needs of specific plants or garden sections. This targeted approach promotes healthier plant growth and mitigates the risk of nutrient runoff, a common issue in densely populated urban settings.

Data-Driven Gardening: Making Informed Decisions

The cornerstone of smart gardening lies in its ability to provide actionable insights derived from data. Gardening apps and sensors collect vast information, from soil conditions and water usage to plant growth patterns and weather impacts. By analyzing this data, urban gardeners can make informed decisions that enhance the health and productivity of their gardens. For example, data on sunlight exposure can help in rearranging plants to maximize photosynthesis, while temperature data can guide the timing of planting and harvesting, ensuring that these activities are conducted under optimal conditions.

Moreover, data analytics can help predict garden trends and potential problems before they become apparent. Predictive analytics can forecast pest invasions based on climate conditions and historical data, allowing for preemptive action to protect plants. Similarly, machine learning algorithms can analyze plant growth over time, identifying patterns that might indicate nutrient deficiencies or other issues. This proactive approach to garden management helps maintain the garden's health, reduces waste, and increases the overall success rate of urban gardening endeavors.

Benefits of Technology: Enhancing Garden Viability and Sustainability

The integration of technology into gardening practice brings myriad benefits, paramount among them being the conservation of resources and the maximization of space, which are two critical considerations in urban environments. Smart gardening technologies help in precisely allocating water and nutrients, conserving these valuable resources and reducing the environmental footprint of gardening. The ability to control and monitor garden conditions remotely adds a layer of convenience and accessibility, encouraging more individuals to take up gardening. This accessibility is crucial in urban settings where traditional gardening knowledge might be limited.

The increased plant survival rates attributable to technological interventions ensure that even beginners can achieve successful harvests, promoting a more sustainable and self-sufficient lifestyle. Moreover, the data collected through smart gardening practices provide invaluable insights into urban agricultural methods, contributing to broader environmental science and urban planning disciplines. These insights can guide future developments in urban gardening, making it more efficient, productive, and integrated into the fabric of city living.

As urban populations continue to grow and the demand for green, sustainable practices increases, leveraging technology in gardening offers a pathway to beautify city spaces and contribute to the ecological and social well-being of urban environments. Thus, smart gardening stands at the forefront of modern urban agriculture, embodying the fusion of nature and technology in creating sustainable, productive, and accessible garden spaces.

Setting up a Simple Drip Irrigation System for Containers

DIY Drip Irrigation Basics: Crafting an Efficient Watering Solution

In the urban garden, where every drop of water counts, setting up a simple drip irrigation system for your container plants can be a game-changer. This system delivers water directly to the base of your plants at a controlled, slow rate, ensuring that every drop is effectively utilized, reducing waste and minimizing evaporation. To begin, you will need a main supply line (usually a thin tubing), a timer (for automation), drip emitters, and tubing connectors. Start by laying out your main supply line along your containers. Use a punch tool to make holes at intervals matching the plant locations. Into each hole, insert a drip emitter. These emitters are crucial as they control the water flow, ensuring each plant receives the right amount based on specific needs. Connect each emitter with a smaller tubing line leading directly to the base of each plant. Finally, attach the main line to a water source. If your setup is extensive, consider using a pressure regulator to maintain a consistent flow and prevent any potential damage to the system due to high water pressure. If you do not have a water source, consider using a 55-gallon drum.

For urban gardeners, the appeal of this system lies not only in its efficiency but also in its adaptability. Drip irrigation can be tailored to fit any container layout and can be expanded or modified as your garden grows or changes. This customization ensures that as you introduce new plants or rearrange your space, your irrigation system can easily adapt, continuing to provide precise watering without extensive overhauls or increased water consumption.

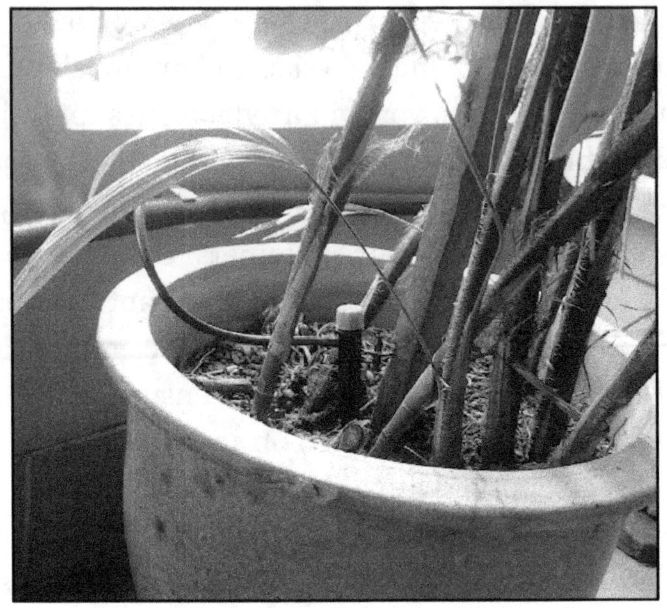

Detail of container irrigation system

Water Efficiency: Maximizing Every Drop

The efficiency of drip irrigation is particularly evident in its ability to minimize water wastage, a critical consideration in urban settings. By delivering water directly to the root zone of each plant, drip systems prevent the common issues of runoff and evaporation that are typical with traditional watering methods like overhead sprinklers. This targeted watering approach is especially beneficial in hot or dry climates where water conservation is paramount. In such environments, the slow and steady drip ensures that water penetrates deeply into the soil, reaching the roots without saturating the surface unnecessarily, which often leads to evaporation.

Automation Options: Simplifying Garden Maintenance

Automating your drip irrigation system can transform your gardening experience by reducing the daily time investment required for plant care. With the integration of a timer, the system can operate on a schedule that suits the specific needs of your plants, delivering water at optimal times without the need for manual intervention. For urban gardeners who juggle busy schedules, this automation ensures that plants receive consistent care, even in the gardener's absence.

For those looking to enhance their system further, integrating a smart water controller offers an advanced level of automation. These smart controllers can adjust watering based on real-time weather conditions by reducing water output on rainy days and increasing it during dry spells. By connecting to local weather stations or using in-built weather sensors, these devices ensure that your garden's watering schedule is responsive and intelligent, adapting to environmental changes with precision and efficiency.

Water Conservation Tips: Cultivating Responsibility

Conserving water in urban gardening is about efficiency and adopting practices that support sustainable water use. One way to enhance the conservation capabilities of your drip irrigation system is to integrate rain barrels. These barrels can collect rainwater, which can then be used to fill your irrigation system's reservoir, reducing your reliance on municipal water systems and using a free, natural resource. When setting up your system, consider the placement of your containers to maximize rain exposure, thereby increasing the amount of water your rain barrels can capture.

Adjusting your system to the specific water needs of different plants is another crucial strategy for conserving water. Use adjustable emitters that allow you to customize the flow rate based on individual plant requirements. This customization means that water-loving plants can receive more frequent or voluminous watering, while succulents or other drought-tolerant plants receive less, ensuring that each plant receives just what it needs without excess.

Maintenance and Adjustments: Ensuring Peak Performance

Maintaining your drip irrigation system is essential for ensuring its longevity and effectiveness. Regularly check for leaks or blockages in the tubing and emitters. Leaks can lead to water wastage, while blockages can prevent water from reaching the plants, potentially stressing or killing them. Cleaning the system, particularly the filters and emitters, at the start and end of each growing season can prevent buildup and damage, extending the system's life.

Regular adjustments may also be necessary as your garden grows and evolves. As plants mature, their water needs can change, and the system should be adjusted accordingly. This might mean changing the placement of emitters, adjusting the flow rates, or even expanding the system to accommodate new plants or containers. By closely monitoring plant health and system performance, you can make timely adjustments that keep your garden thriving and your water usage optimized.

In urban gardening, where every resource counts, setting up a simple drip irrigation system provides a reliable and efficient way to ensure your plants thrive. By following these guidelines, you can create a system that saves time, conserves water, and grows healthy plants, all while contributing to a more sustainable urban environment. With these tools at your disposal, your garden can become a source of joy and beauty and a testament to responsible and efficient gardening practices.

Advanced Composting Techniques for Small Spaces

Composting offers a remarkable solution for waste reduction and soil enhancement in constrained urban living environments. Despite limited outdoor space, urban gardeners can adopt efficient composting methods such as bokashi bins and worm composting, techniques well-suited to small-scale operations. These methods facilitate the recycling of kitchen scraps into valuable compost and enrich urban gardening experiences, contributing to sustainable living practices.

Composting Methods: Adapting to Urban Constraints

The bokashi method, originating from Japanese practices, utilizes an anaerobic process that ferments organic waste in sealed containers. This method is particularly advantageous for apartment dwellers due to its odorless nature and the speed at which it converts waste into compost. The bokashi method accelerates decomposition by introducing effective microorganisms (EM) to the organic matter in airtight containers, preventing the typical smell associated with composting. This method is versatile, accepting a range of kitchen waste, including items traditionally not recommended for open compost systems, such as cooked foods and dairy products.

Worm composting, or vermicomposting, is another excellent option for indoor composting. This method uses red wiggler worms to break down organic waste into high-quality compost, which is suitable for enriching potting mixes or adding nutrients to your plants. The process is carried out in bins that can be stored under sinks, closets, or any other small space available within an urban home. Worm composting not only processes waste efficiently but also produces worm tea, a nutrient-rich liquid fertilizer that can be used to boost plant growth.

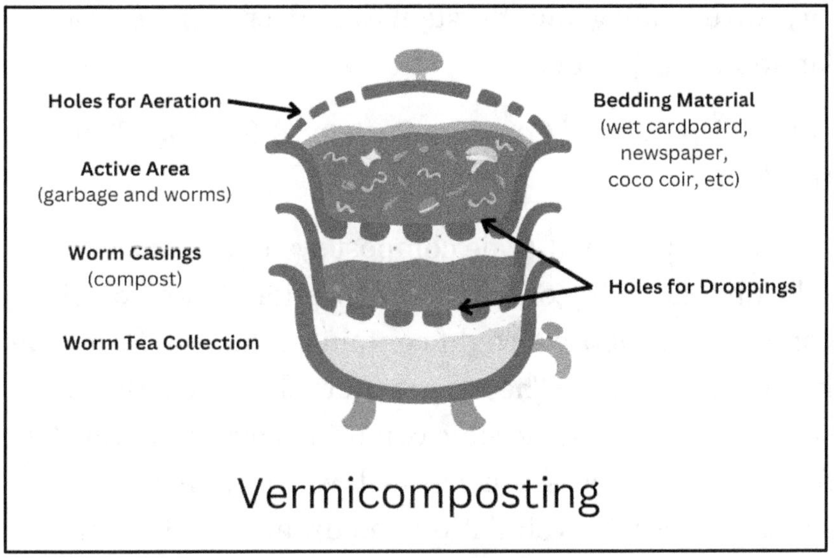

Detail of a vermicompost setup

Benefits of Homemade Compost: Enhancing Urban Soil

Creating your own compost in an urban setting is immensely beneficial, transforming organic waste into a resource that significantly improves soil health. Compost adds essential nutrients back into the soil, promoting healthier plant growth and increased resilience against pests and diseases. Moreover, it improves soil structure, enhancing aeration and water retention, which are crucial for plant roots to develop fully. Using homemade compost reduces reliance on commercial fertilizers, many of which come with environmental costs due to their production and transportation. Furthermore, composting contributes to municipal waste reduction, lessening the burden on city waste management systems and decreasing overall landfill contributions.

Setting Up a Small Compost System: A Step-by-Step Guide

Establishing a small-scale compost system begins with selecting the right container and location. For bokashi composting, choose airtight containers that can fit in your kitchen or balcony. These containers should be easy to seal to ensure the anaerobic conditions necessary for the fermentation process. In contrast, worm composting requires bins with ventilation and drainage to keep the worms alive and active. These bins can be commercially purchased or handcrafted from plastic containers by adding drainage holes and a tap for draining worm tea.

Once your container is ready, the next step involves layering your organic waste with bokashi bran or bedding material for the worms. For bokashi, alternate layers of kitchen waste with bokashi bran, pressing down each layer to remove air pockets and seal the container tightly after each addition. In worm composting, start with bedding made from shredded newspaper or cardboard, moistened to provide a welcoming environment for the worms. Add your worms, and gradually add your kitchen scraps, burying them under the bedding to avoid attracting pests.

Maintaining Your Compost: Ensuring Effective Decomposition

Proper maintenance is crucial for the success of your composting efforts. In bokashi composting, regularly drain the liquid that accumulates at the bottom of the container to prevent spoilage of the compost. This bokashi tea can be diluted and used as a plant liquid fertilizer. Once the container is full, seal it and let it sit for two to three weeks to complete the fermentation process. Afterward, the contents can be buried in soil to finish decomposing or added to a traditional compost pile to integrate into the compost fully.

In worm composting, balance green (nitrogen-rich) and brown (carbon-rich) materials to ensure rapid decomposition and prevent odors. Keep the bedding moist but not wet and regularly check that the bin's temperature remains conducive to worm activity, ideally between 55- and 77-degrees Fahrenheit. Harvest the compost every few months by separating the worms from the compost and restarting the bin with fresh bedding.

These advanced composting techniques empower urban gardeners to contribute positively to environmental sustainability while enhancing their gardening practices. By transforming kitchen waste into nutrient-rich compost, you enrich your plants and partake in a cycle of renewal that benefits the urban ecosystem. As we continue exploring sustainable practices in urban gardening, these waste reduction and resource reclamation methods stand as testaments to the innovative spirit of urban green spaces.

As we wrap up this exploration of advanced composting techniques, we prepare to delve deeper into the world of sustainable urban gardening practices in the following chapters. The journey of transforming your limited urban space into a productive and sustainable green area continues with further insights and strategies that enhance your gardening experience and contribute to a healthier urban environment.

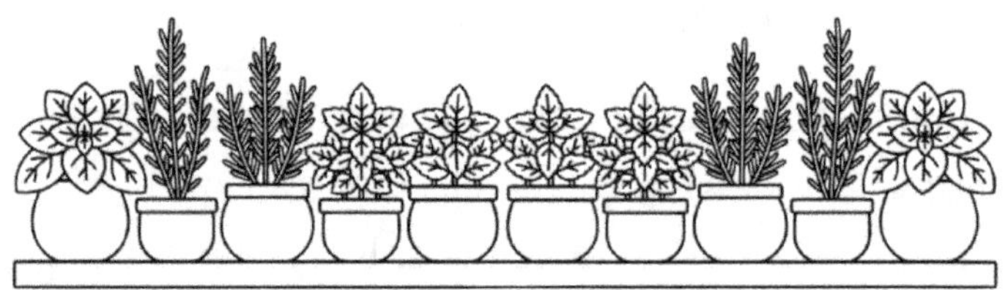

Key Chapter 7 Takeaways:

- Use hydroponic systems (starting with simple wick setups) to grow plants efficiently without soil while conserving space and water.

- Explore aquaponics as a closed-loop system that supports both plants and fish through natural nutrient cycling.

- Leverage smart gardening tools (sensors, automation, apps) to reduce guesswork, save time, and improve plant survival.

- Install a simple drip irrigation system to deliver water directly to roots, conserve water, and automate consistent care.
- Recycle kitchen waste into plant nutrition with bokashi or vermicomposting, creating rich compost and liquid fertilizer in small spaces.

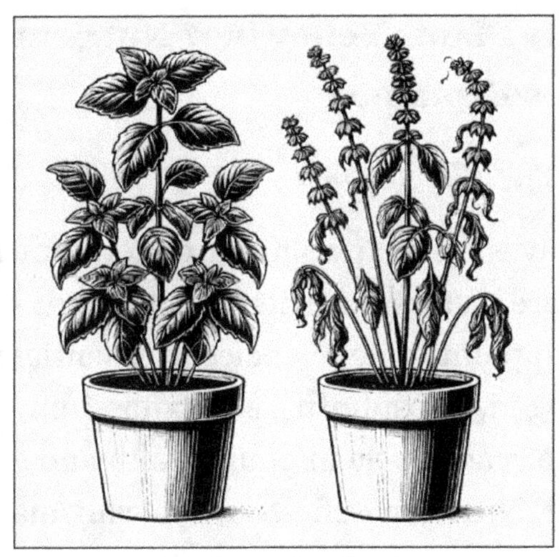

Chapter 8: Troubleshooting Common Container Gardening Issues

In container gardening, encountering challenges is a part of the growth process, both for the plants and the gardener. Urban dwellers often face unique hurdles due to restricted growing conditions. Yet these obstacles should not deter you. Instead, they invite an opportunity to deepen your understanding and refine your gardening skills. This chapter focuses on diagnosing and resolving one of the most puzzling issues you might encounter: unexplained yellowing of plant leaves, often a telltale sign of nutrient deficiencies. By mastering identifying and correcting these deficiencies, you ensure your plants survive and thrive in their urban environment.

Why Are My Plants Yellowing? Nutrient Deficiencies Explained

Signs of Nutrient Deficiency

Yellowing leaves can alarm any gardener, indicating that your plants are distressed. This symptom, known as chlorosis, can point to deficiencies in essential nutrients such as nitrogen, phosphorus, and potassium, each of which plays a crucial role in plant health and development. Nitrogen deficiency typically manifests as a general yellowing of older leaves as the nutrient is mobilized to new growth. In contrast, phosphorus deficiency often causes older leaves to exhibit a dark green hue before progressing to a purple or reddish color. Potassium deficiency appears as yellowing at the leaf edges, progressing inward, coupled with brown scorching and curling.

These visual cues serve as critical signals prompting immediate action to rectify nutrient imbalances. Understanding these signs is essential, as they help pinpoint the deficiencies affecting your plants and guide targeted corrective measures.

Correcting Deficiencies

Addressing nutrient deficiencies begins with choosing the right type of fertilizer. Organic options such as fish emulsion or compost can provide a balanced supply of essential nutrients, promoting healthy growth without the risk of chemical buildup that can occur with synthetic fertilizers. Following recommended rates and methods is crucial when applying fertilizer to avoid over-fertilization, which can harm plant roots and exacerbate nutrient imbalances.

For nitrogen deficiency, incorporating a high-nitrogen organic fertilizer or adding composted manure can help restore your plants' vibrant green color. Bone meal is an effective organic option for phosphorus-poor plants that can enhance root development and flowering. In the case of potassium deficiency, kelp meal or sulfate of potash are viable organic amendments that can strengthen plant resistance to disease and environmental stress.

Soil Testing

Conducting a soil test is advisable before adjusting your fertilization routine. This diagnostic tool provides a detailed analysis of the soil's nutrient content, pH level, and other properties crucial for plant health. Soil testing kits are readily available at garden centers and online, offering an accessible way for urban gardeners to gain insights into their soil's condition without guessing. By understanding the specific nutrient needs of your soil, you can tailor your fertilization practices more precisely, ensuring that your plants receive exactly what they need for optimal growth.

Preventive Nutrition

Preventive measures are vital in maintaining the ongoing health of your garden. Regular, balanced feeding, aligned with your plants' specific growth stages and needs, helps prevent nutrient deficiencies before they start. Incorporating organic compost into your soil mix improves soil structure and water retention and provides a slow-release source of nutrients, enhancing soil fertility sustainably. This proactive approach to nutrition helps create a resilient garden ecosystem where plants can thrive despite the challenges posed by urban container environments. Learn more about the detailed signs of nutrition deficiencies including symptoms, ways to identify them, and simple fixes in APPENDIX 6 starting on page 250. Three of the most common deficiencies are:

- Nitrogen (N): Older leaves turn yellow; stunted growth.
- Phosphorus (P): Dark green leaves turning purplish; stunted growth and poor flowering.
- Potassium (K): Yellowing at leaf edges; brown spots and curled margins.

Understanding and addressing nutrient deficiencies in container gardening requires a balanced approach of careful observation, targeted nutrition, and regular soil health assessments. By equipping yourself with the knowledge to recognize and correct these deficiencies, you enhance your ability to maintain a healthy, vibrant urban garden. This proactive management ensures your plants survive and flourish, bringing life and beauty to your urban space. As you continue to nurture your garden, remember that each challenge you overcome adds to your growing experience, transforming you into a more skilled and confident gardener.

Overcoming Root-Bound Plants: Signs and Solutions

In the compact realm of urban container gardening, managing the spatial needs of rapidly growing plants presents a challenge that, if not addressed timely, can lead to the issue of root bounding. This phenomenon occurs when the roots of a plant grow to the extent that they have no room left to expand within the confines of their container, leading to several growth and health issues for the plant. Recognizing the signs of a root-bound plant is crucial in taking proactive measures to alleviate this stressor. Typical indications include noticeably stunted growth despite adequate care, roots emerging excessively from the drainage holes, or, when visible, a dense web of roots that seems to take over the soil space. Additionally, you might observe that water runs straight through the pot without being retained, indicating that dense roots are displacing the soil.

Addressing a root-bound situation begins with careful repotting. To repot a root-bound plant, prepare a larger container with the appropriate potting mix, which should be rich in nutrients and well-draining. Gently remove the plant from its current container, which may require tapping or breaking the pot if the roots are tightly bound. Once removed, examine the root ball. If the roots have formed a tight spiral around the perimeter, they must be loosened to encourage outward growth. Using your fingers or a sterile knife, gently tease the roots apart. If they are exceptionally dense, making a few vertical cuts in the root mass can help stimulate new root growth. Place the plant in the new pot and fill it with fresh potting mix, tamping down lightly to eliminate large air pockets, and thoroughly water to settle the roots.

Root pruning can be an interim solution when immediate repotting isn't feasible. This involves removing the plant from its container and pruning away a portion of the overgrown roots. This should be done carefully, removing no more than one-third of the root mass with clean, sharp cuts. This method can temporarily alleviate the stress on the plant by reducing the demand on its root system, allowing it to maintain health until a more suitable time for repotting. However, it's a stopgap measure and should not substitute for eventually providing the plant with a more spacious environment.

Preventing plants from becoming root-bound is preferable to addressing the after-effects. Selecting the right container size plays a pivotal role in prevention. As a rule, when choosing a new pot, opt for one that is one to two inches larger in diameter than the current pot for smaller plants and up to four inches for larger plants. This provides enough space for roots to grow without being excessive, which could lead to waterlogging issues. Monitoring your plants' growth and being mindful of their typical root development patterns can help you anticipate when a pot upgrade is necessary. Regularly lifting the plant to check for emerging roots can also be a practical monitoring method.

Incorporating these strategies into your gardening routine helps mitigate the risk of your plants becoming root-bound, ensuring they remain healthy and vibrant. By understanding the signs of root constriction and knowing how to address them effectively, you empower yourself to maintain the well-being of your container garden, fostering a lush and thriving green space amidst the urban landscape.

Addressing Waterlogging and Poor Drainage in Containers

In urban container gardening, managing water effectively is crucial, not just for the plant's survival but for its thriving. One common issue is waterlogging, which can severely impact plant health, leading to stunted growth and potentially fatal root diseases. Waterlogging typically results from a few critical oversights: improper container choice, inadequate drainage provision, and the use of overly compacted soil. Each of these factors contributes to an environment where water accumulates around the plant roots more than it should, drowning them and cutting off their air supply.

Containers without sufficient drainage holes or those made from materials that do not allow water to pass through easily can trap water inside, leading to saturated soil conditions. Similarly, using garden soil or a very dense potting mix can hinder water movement, causing the lower layers of the soil to become waterlogged even if the surface appears dry. It's vital to select the correct type of container with adequate drainage holes and use a potting mix specifically designed for container gardening, which typically includes a combination of peat, perlite, and vermiculite to ensure good drainage and aeration.

To correct existing drainage issues, start by assessing the situation thoroughly. If your plants show signs of stress due to poor drainage and you confirm the soil is excessively wet, consider repotting them into a more suitable container with proper drainage holes. If repotting is not immediately feasible, try to improve the situation by gently lifting the plant and inserting additional materials like gravel or Styrofoam pieces at the base of the container to enhance water flow. Adding these materials can help create a drainage layer that keeps the roots from sitting in water, thereby preventing the anaerobic conditions that lead to root rot.

Signs of Water Stress

Recognizing the signs of water stress associated with poor drainage is key to taking timely action to save affected plants. Initial symptoms often include yellowing leaves, a telltale sign that is mistakenly attributed solely to nutrient deficiencies. However, in the case of waterlogging, a general limpness in the plant accompanies this yellowing, and the soil may emit a foul odor, indicative of root decay. Other signs include leaf drop, mold growth on the soil's surface, and roots that appear brown and mushy when inspected. Identifying these signs early can make the difference between rescuing a plant and losing it to decay.

Rescue and Recovery

Rescuing a waterlogged plant involves a careful approach to avoid further stressing the plant. Begin by gently removing the plant from its container to assess the extent of the damage. Examine the roots carefully. Healthy roots should appear white and firm, not slimy or dark. Trim away any rotten roots with a clean, sharp pair of scissors or pruning shears, as these cannot be revived and will only spread decay if left in place. After pruning the damaged roots, repot the plant in fresh, well-draining potting mix, ensuring the container has adequate drainage holes. If the original container is to be reused, clean it thoroughly to remove any lingering pathogens or debris that could harm the plant upon reintroduction.

Water recovery should be gradual; after repotting, water lightly to settle the soil around the roots and wait until the top inch of soil is dry before watering again. This cautious approach ensures the plant has adequate moisture without risking further waterlogging. Monitoring the plant over the following weeks is crucial to ensure it is recovering well and not showing further signs of stress.

Addressing waterlogging and improving drainage are not merely reactive measures but should be integrated into your regular gardening practices. Ensuring that every container has sufficient drainage, choosing the right soil mix, and being cautious with watering schedules are all proactive steps that help prevent the occurrence of waterlogging. By understanding the causes and implementing these strategies, you empower yourself to maintain the health and vigor of your urban garden, ensuring that your plants remain robust and flourishing in their container environments.

Reviving Drought-Stressed Plants in Urban Gardens

Drought stress in urban gardens is a prevalent issue that can dramatically affect plant health, growth, and productivity. Early identification of drought stress is vital to mitigate its impact and ensure the survival of your plants. Typically, the initial signs of drought stress include wilting, the plant's response to insufficient water intake affecting its rigidity. Leaves may appear droopy and feel soft to the touch. Another common symptom is the dryness of the leaves, which often feel brittle or crispy, accompanied by a dull, faded coloration rather than their usual vibrant green. Growth may also slow down noticeably as the plant conserves its resources, focusing on survival rather than expansion. Observing these signs early allows immediate intervention, crucial for the plant's recovery and continued health.

Immediate remedial actions are essential upon noticing signs of drought stress. The primary goal is to rehydrate the plant without causing additional stress from sudden overwatering. Begin by gently watering the plant using a slow and steady method, such as drip irrigation or a watering can with a small spout to mimic natural rainfall. This method helps the soil absorb moisture more effectively without causing runoff, which is common when the soil is dry and hardened. If the soil is extremely dry, consider lightly aerating it with a fork before watering to enhance moisture penetration. It's also beneficial to temporarily relocate the plant to a shaded area if it's typically exposed to full sun, reducing evaporation rates and giving it a better chance to absorb and retain moisture.

Adjusting your regular watering practices is crucial to prevent future drought stress. Implementing a consistent watering schedule tailored to the specific needs of your plants, considering factors such as species, life stage, and current weather conditions, is essential. Setting up self-watering containers can be an effective solution in urban settings where daily natural watering isn't feasible. These systems ensure that plants have a consistent moisture supply, drawing water as needed through wicking systems that connect the plant's root zone with a water reservoir. Additionally, applying a layer of organic mulch around your plants can significantly help retain soil moisture by reducing surface evaporation and providing a barrier against wind and sun drying effects.

Building resilience against occasional drought involves enhancing the overall health of your plants through careful soil management and appropriate watering techniques. Deep watering practices, which involve infrequent but thorough watering sessions, encourage plants to develop deeper root systems, making them more capable of accessing water from lower soil levels during dry periods. This method is preferable to frequent shallow watering, which promotes shallow root growth, making plants more vulnerable to drought. Improving soil structure by incorporating organic matter such as compost also plays a crucial role. This improves water retention and enhances soil fertility, supporting robust plant growth that can better withstand adverse conditions.

By employing these strategies, you empower yourself to effectively manage drought stress in your urban garden, ensuring that your plants survive and thrive despite the challenges posed by their environment. This proactive approach to garden management underscores the importance of understanding and responding to the specific needs of your plants, fostering a lush and productive garden that enhances your urban living space.

Wind Protection for High-Rise Balcony Gardens

High-rise balcony gardens offer unique challenges due to their exposure to elements, particularly wind, which can be both a subtle breeze and a disruptive gale. The increased elevation often subjects these gardens to stronger winds than those experienced at ground level, leading to potential issues such as rapid dehydration of plants and physical damage ranging from torn leaves to broken stems. Wind can also cause significant soil erosion, disturbing the root systems and ultimately affecting the overall health and stability of the plants. Understanding these challenges is crucial for maintaining a thriving balcony garden amidst the gusty conditions typical of high altitudes.

Creating effective windbreaks is an essential strategy to mitigate the effects of wind. Windbreaks reduce wind speed and deflect the flow away from sensitive plants, thereby lessening the physical stress experienced by the garden. One practical solution is fabric or fine mesh screens, which can be installed around the balcony's perimeter. These materials are particularly effective as they cut down on wind intensity without completely blocking light, thus maintaining essential conditions for photosynthesis. Another robust option involves the installation of trellises, which can serve dual purposes: reducing wind impact and supporting climbing plants or vines that, once mature, can act as additional natural wind barriers.

Strategically placing taller plants or shrubs in containers can also serve as wind blocks for more sensitive understory plants. For instance, placing potted small trees or large shrubs upwind will shield smaller, more vulnerable species from the brunt of the wind. When arranging these plants, it is crucial to ensure that they are wind-tolerant to prevent their own foliage from damage. Additionally, the layout should be planned so that these taller plants do not cast excessive shade on smaller plants requiring abundant sunlight.

Choosing Wind-Resistant Plants

When selecting flora for a wind-prone balcony garden, choosing plants naturally resistant to wind stress will significantly increase the garden's resilience and ease of maintenance. Such plants typically feature flexible stems and leaves that can bend rather than break under the force of the wind, and they often have a more compact growth habit to resist being uprooted. Grasses like Miscanthus or Festuca are excellent for windy areas due to their flexible leaves and strong root systems. Hardy shrubs like Juniper and Boxwood can also perform well, providing structure and protection. These plants survive in windy conditions and can thrive, adding movement and texture to the garden while serving as organic windbreaks.

Container Stabilization

Securing containers is another critical aspect of maintaining a high-rise balcony garden. Unsecured pots can be hazardous in strong winds, posing risks not just to the plants they contain but also potentially causing damage to property or injury to individuals below. To counter this, choose containers made from heavy materials such as ceramic or metal that are less likely to tip over. Adding weight at the base, such as with rocks or sand, can enhance stability for lighter containers. Additionally, grouping pots closely together can help distribute the wind load among them, reducing the chance of individual pots tipping. For added security, consider using ties or brackets to anchor containers directly to the balcony railing or walls, ensuring they remain in place even in strong winds.

Implementing these strategies effectively transforms the challenge of wind into an accounted-for factor in your gardening plans, allowing you to cultivate a high-rise balcony garden that is both beautiful and resilient. By understanding and adapting to the specific demands of your environment, you can create a green space that not only survives but thrives, bringing life and beauty to the urban skyline. These measures ensure that your garden remains a safe, enjoyable, and flourishing haven amidst the gusts and gales characteristic of elevated urban gardening.

Adjusting Plant Care for Microclimates in Urban Areas

Understanding the concept of microclimates is pivotal for urban gardeners, as it illuminates the subtle yet significant environmental variations that can exist even within relatively small geographical areas. A microclimate refers to the localized climate that differs from the surrounding areas; within an urban setting, these can be influenced by factors such as proximity to buildings, bodies of water, concrete surfaces, and other infrastructure elements. These structures can significantly alter temperatures, light exposure, humidity levels, and wind patterns within a confined space. For instance, the north side of a building may receive significantly less sunlight than the south side, and areas near large concrete surfaces may experience higher temperatures due to heat retention.

Observing and identifying these microclimates within your gardening space is the first step in effectively adapting your plant care strategies. Begin by spending time in your garden space throughout the day, noting areas that receive more shade, wind, or sun. Keeping track of how these conditions change with the seasons is crucial for long-term planning. Tools such as thermometers and humidity sensors can provide more precise data about these conditions. Once you understand the different microclimates around your garden, selecting plants becomes more informed. Opt for species that naturally thrive under each specific set of conditions. For example, ferns and hostas might prosper in the cooler, shaded areas, while sun-loving plants like lavender and rosemary will thrive in the brighter, warmer spots.

Customizing care for your plants according to their microclimates involves more than just appropriate plant selection; it extends to tailored watering, feeding, and general care routines. For instance, evaporation rates might be higher in warmer microclimates, necessitating more frequent watering to ensure plants remain hydrated. Conversely, the risk of overwatering increases in cooler or shaded areas as soil retains moisture for longer periods. These conditions require reducing watering frequency to prevent issues such as root rot. Similarly, feeding schedules should be adjusted based on the plant's exposure to sunlight and its resultant growth rate. For example, plants in high-light areas may require more frequent feeding to support faster growth than their counterparts in shaded areas.

Protection and adaptation strategies are crucial for mitigating adverse effects caused by challenging urban microclimates. In areas exposed to intense sunlight reflected off windows or metallic surfaces, installing shading cloth during the hottest parts of the day can prevent leaf scorch. For plants in windy corridors, often found between tall buildings, windbreaks such as trellis panels can reduce wind intensity, minimizing dehydration and physical damage to the plants. Furthermore, gradually acclimating new plants to these conditions can increase their resilience. Start by placing them in the intended location for short periods each day, gradually increasing their exposure until they are accustomed to the new environment. This process helps strengthen their tolerance to specific microclimatic conditions, enhancing overall plant health and longevity.

Incorporating these microclimate-specific strategies into your gardening practice improves the health and appearance of your garden and increases its ecological efficiency. By aligning your gardening techniques with the natural environment, you reduce the need for interventions like excessive watering or chemical use, promoting a more sustainable urban gardening practice. This thoughtful approach to urban gardening underscores the importance of understanding and respecting the natural environmental variations, leading to a more successful and rewarding gardening experience.

As this chapter on adjusting plant care for urban microclimates concludes, we reflect on the importance of detailed observation and tailored care in overcoming the unique challenges posed by urban gardening. The insights gained here enhance your immediate gardening efforts and contribute to a broader understanding of environmental stewardship and sustainability. Looking ahead, the next chapter will explore further innovative strategies in urban gardening, continuing to expand your toolkit for cultivating a thriving garden in the heart of the city.

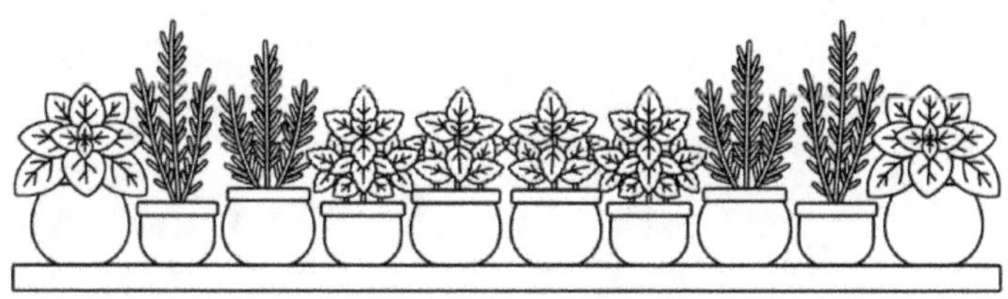

Key Chapter 8 Takeaways:

- Use leaf color and growth patterns to distinguish nutrient deficiencies from watering or drainage problems before making corrections.

- Prevent and correct root-bound plants by monitoring root growth, repotting on time, and loosening roots during transplanting.

- Avoid waterlogging by choosing containers with proper drainage, using container-specific soil, and adjusting watering habits.

- Restore drought-stressed plants gradually with slow rehydration, shade, mulch, and deeper watering practices.

- Protect balcony gardens from environmental stress by managing wind exposure, container stability, and microclimates with thoughtful plant placement and care adjustments.

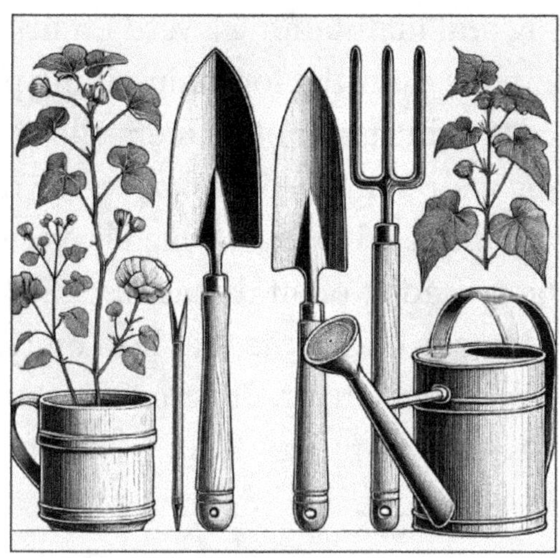

Chapter 9: Essential Tools and Resources

The Essential Container Gardening Toolkit

Navigating the labyrinth of gardening tools available on the market can be daunting and confusing, especially for the urban gardener grappling with limited space constraints and the ambitions of a burgeoning green thumb. This section is dedicated to distilling the options down to the quintessential toolkit necessary for every container gardener. Mastery of your garden begins with the right tools, which enhance your gardening efficiency and elevate your experience from mundane to magical.

Tool Selection: The Foundation of Gardening Success

At the heart of container gardening lies a suite of indispensable tools, each serving a unique purpose that aids in creating and maintaining a verdant urban oasis. Firstly, pruners are essential for maintaining plant health and aesthetics. A robust pair of pruners allows you to precisely shape your plants, control overgrowth, and remove dead or diseased foliage, which is crucial in preventing the spread of plant diseases. Choose bypass pruners, which make clean cuts that heal quickly, over anvil-style pruners, which tend to crush the stems, potentially harming the plant.

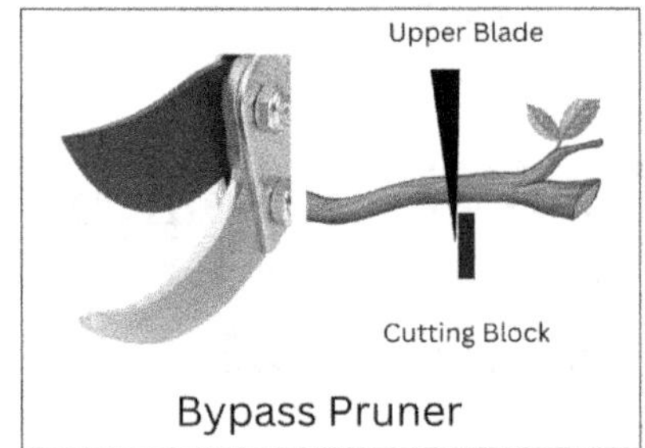

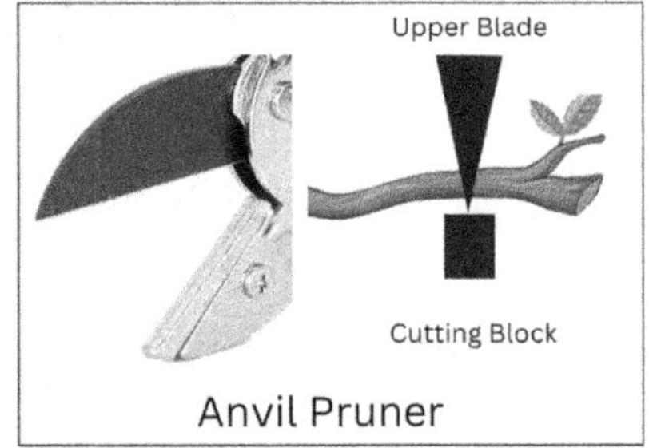

Detail of bypass pruner vs anvil pruner

Next, a gardener should have a reliable watering can. Choose one with a long spout to ensure a gentle flow of water, minimizing disturbance to the soil while accurately targeting the roots where water is most needed. A watering can with a detachable rose (the sprinkler-like head) is particularly versatile, offering different watering options for seedlings and mature plants.

A soil scoop, often overlooked, is another vital tool in the container gardener's arsenal. Larger and sturdier than a typical garden trowel, a soil scoop is perfectly shaped for transplanting, mixing soil amendments, and filling pots with soil. Its broad, deep basin allows for efficient work with minimal spillage, which is particularly beneficial when working within the confined spaces of an urban garden.

Tool Care: Prolonging the Life of Your Gardening Investments

Maintaining your gardening tools is not merely about cleanliness; it's about extending the life of your investments and ensuring they remain effective and safe to use. Regular cleaning to remove soil and plant debris, followed by thorough drying, is essential to prevent rust and deterioration. Tools should be stored in a dry environment to avoid moisture damage. Sharpening your tools, particularly pruners and shears, ensures they deliver optimal performance and make clean cuts that promote plant health. A simple sharpening stone or file can be used periodically to maintain sharp edges.

Ergonomic Tools: Enhancing Comfort and Accessibility

Ergonomics is pivotal in selecting gardening tools, especially for urban dwellers facing physical constraints such as limited space or mobility issues. Ergonomically designed tools are crafted to reduce strain on your body, minimizing the risk of injury and fatigue. Tools with padded handles, lightweight materials, and designs that naturally complement the movement of your body can significantly enhance your gardening comfort. For gardeners with arthritis or hand strength issues, ergonomic tools with easy grip handles or those designed for minimal force usage can be particularly beneficial, allowing gardening to be a joy rather than a chore.

Storage Solutions: Keeping Your Tools Organized and Accessible

Efficient storage solutions are integral to managing your gardening tools, particularly in an urban setting where space is at a premium. Creative storage options include hanging organizers mounted on walls or over doors, magnetic strips for metal tools, and specially designed racks installed in small sheds, closets and/or balconies. Proper organization saves space and keeps your tools conveniently accessible, making your gardening more productive and enjoyable. Consider labeling compartments and hooks, ensuring that each tool has a designated place, which aids in maintaining order and ensuring that no tool goes misplaced.

Equipping yourself with the essential tools of the trade, caring for them properly, and storing them efficiently set the stage for a successful and enjoyable gardening experience. These tools become extensions of your gardening intentions, transforming your urban space into a flourishing green retreat that offers sustenance and sanctuary.

Books and Guides for the Avid Reader Container Gardener

The value of a well-curated library cannot be overstated in the quest to cultivate a thriving container garden within the confines of urban spaces. Books and guides serve as repositories of gardening wisdom and as sources of inspiration and practical advice. For the urban gardener, particularly those navigating the nuances of container gardening, selecting the right reading material can significantly enhance understanding and success. This section introduces essential readings covering a broad spectrum of gardening topics, each catering to different aspects of container gardening, and ranging from fundamental principles to specialized practices. Learn more about gardening books in Appendix 8 on page 258.

Foundational Texts: Building Your Gardening Knowledge Base

Foundational texts are indispensable for readers beginning their journey into container gardening. These books provide a solid grounding in the basic principles of gardening in containers, offering insight into everything from selecting the correct soil and containers to understanding plant needs and watering techniques. A quintessential read in this category is *"The Vegetable Gardener's Container Bible"* by Edward C. Smith. This guide demystifies growing vegetables in containers, offering clear, concise information invaluable for beginners. It covers soil composition and container selection and provides a comprehensive guide to growing common vegetables, making it an indispensable resource for those looking to grow their food in limited spaces.

Another invaluable resource is *"Container Gardening Complete"* by Jessica Walliser. This book is a treasure trove of information, covering the how-to of planting and maintaining container gardens and delving into the aesthetics of arranging them beautifully. Its detailed discussions on container types, suitable plant varieties, and decorative tips make it an excellent guide for ensuring health and visual appeal in urban garden spaces.

Specialized Topics: Enhancing Your Gardening Expertise

As your confidence and experience grow, delving into more specialized topics can help expand your gardening repertoire. For urban gardeners interested in edible gardening, *"Grow All You Can Eat in Three Square Feet"* offers innovative solutions to space constraints, demonstrating how various vegetables and herbs can be grown in surprisingly small areas. This book is particularly useful for apartment dwellers looking to maximize their balcony or windowsill spaces for edible gardening.

On the ornamental front, *"Container Gardening for All Seasons"* by Barbara Wise provides information on creating year-round visual interest through container gardens. It offers unique plant suggestions and design ideas that keep your space vibrant across different seasons, which is crucial in maintaining an engaging and dynamic urban garden.

Pam Penick's *"The Water-Saving Garden"* is essential for those committed to environmentally sustainable practices. It focuses on techniques and plant choices that minimize water usage, which is a critical consideration in urban areas where water conservation is increasingly prioritized. This book is particularly pertinent for gardeners in drought-prone regions, providing creative ideas for gardening with limited water resources.

Inspirational Books: Sparking Creativity in Urban Gardening

Sometimes, what a gardener needs most is a dose of inspiration to reimagine what's possible in a small space. *"Small-Space Container Gardens"* by Fern Richardson is an inspirational guide to transforming small spaces into vibrant, lush areas. It discusses the practical aspects of container gardening and delves into decorative elements, incorporating art and upcycled materials to create stunning visual displays that reflect personal style and creativity.

Resource Guides: Quick-Reference Tools for Everyday Gardening Challenges

Lastly, no gardener's library is complete without a go-to resource for quick troubleshooting. Pippa Greenwood's

"The Container Gardener's Handbook" perfectly serves this need, offering tips and tricks for dealing with common issues such as pests, diseases, and watering problems. It's easy-to-navigate format makes it an excellent quick-reference guide during busy gardening days or when unexpected problems arise.

Incorporating these books into your gardening practice provides not only the knowledge needed for successful container gardening but also a source of continuous learning and inspiration. As you build your gardening library, each book will guide you through the technical aspects of gardening and inspire you to push creative boundaries, ensuring your small urban space is both a productive and enchanting green retreat.

Must-Have Apps and Websites for Gardeners

In the digital age, gardening has transcended traditional methods, embracing technology to facilitate more efficient and informed gardening practices. For urban gardeners, particularly those new to the craft, navigating the vast array of digital tools available can significantly enhance their gardening experience. This section delves into the essential digital resources that every urban gardener should consider integrating into their gardening repertoire. These tools simplify various gardening tasks and provide a wealth of information, making gardening more accessible and enjoyable. Learn more about gardening websites and apps in Appendix 8 on page 260.

Gardening Apps: Digital Assistants for the Modern Gardener

The convenience of smartphones has brought forth various apps designed to assist gardeners in managing their plant care routines effectively. Essential apps for plant identification, such as PlantNet, allow users to snap a photo of a plant and instantly receive information about its species, care requirements, and more. This tool is invaluable for beginners who may need to become more familiar with the flora in their urban environment. Furthermore, apps like Waterbot and Garden Manager remind you of watering schedules, helping you keep your plants hydrated without the guesswork. These apps can be customized according to each plant's needs, ensuring your urban garden remains lush and healthy.

For those dealing with plant health issues, Plantix offers a robust platform for diagnosing plant diseases and pests. Users receive diagnostic information and treatment suggestions by uploading images of affected plant areas. This app can be particularly beneficial in preventing the spread of diseases in the confined spaces of urban gardens, where such issues can escalate rapidly if not addressed promptly.

Educational Websites: A Gateway to Gardening Wisdom

The internet has websites dedicated to gardening education, offering articles, detailed tutorials, and interactive forums where novice and experienced gardeners can expand their knowledge. Websites like Gardeners' World and The Spruce provide comprehensive articles that cover everything from basic gardening techniques to advanced tips for specific plants. These resources are ideal for self-education, allowing you to learn quickly and delve into topics that interest you the most.

Forums on sites such as GardenWeb and Houzz offer a platform for community interaction where you can pose questions, share experiences, and receive advice from fellow gardeners worldwide. This community aspect can be incredibly supportive for urban gardeners who may not have direct access to gardening clubs or networks in their immediate environment.

Plant Databases: Comprehensive Repositories of Plant Knowledge

Access to accurate and extensive plant information is crucial for successful gardening. Online plant databases such as Missouri Botanical Garden's Plant Finder (www.missouribotanicalgarden.org/PlantFinder) and USDA's PLANTS Database (www.plants.usda.gov) offer detailed profiles of various plant species, including their care requirements, hardiness zones, and growth habits. These databases are particularly useful for urban gardeners who need to understand which plants will thrive in specific conditions, such as limited light or space. By researching plants before purchasing, you can make informed decisions that lead to better plant survival rates and a more satisfying gardening experience.

Design Tools: Visualizing and Planning Your Urban Garden

Finally, the layout and design of your garden can significantly impact its success and aesthetic appeal. Online design tools and apps like Garden Planner and My Garden allow you to digitally visualize and plan your garden space. These tools enable you to experiment with different plant arrangements, container styles, and garden themes without physical effort. This can be particularly useful in maximizing the limited space available in urban environments, allowing for optimal use of every square inch. Whether planning a single container or an entire balcony garden, these design tools offer a user-friendly interface to bring your garden vision to life.

By integrating these digital tools and resources into your gardening practice, you empower yourself with knowledge, streamline your gardening tasks, and enhance your overall gardening experience. The digital age offers unprecedented access to information and community, transforming urban gardening from a solitary pursuit into a connected, enriching activity that brings nature closer to your urban lifestyle. As you continue to explore and utilize these tools, they become not just aids but essential components of your gardening success in the urban jungle.

Local Resources and Communities for Gardeners

The significance of tapping into local resources and communities cannot be overstressed in urban gardening. These networks provide a wealth of knowledge, practical support, and enhanced opportunities for personal and communal growth in gardening proficiency. Engaging with local gardening clubs, nurseries, community gardens, and educational workshops enriches your gardening journey, offering many benefits from collective wisdom and shared experiences. Learn more about local gardening resources in Appendix 8 on page 261.

Gardening Clubs: Networking and Resource Sharing

Joining a local gardening club or society can profoundly impact your gardening approach, offering invaluable networking and resource-sharing avenues. These clubs often serve as a nexus for like-minded individuals eager to exchange knowledge, techniques, and plant cuttings. The collaborative environment fosters a learning culture that can accelerate your gardening skills exponentially. Memberships typically provide access to exclusive seminars, newsletters, and events, all geared toward enhancing your understanding and capabilities in gardening. Moreover, the collective purchasing power of clubs can enable access to high-quality gardening supplies at reduced costs. Engaging with these clubs also offers the emotional and motivational benefits of belonging to a community with shared interests, providing a support network that is particularly beneficial during challenging times in your gardening endeavors.

Nurseries and Garden Centers: Expert Advice and Quality Supplies

Developing relationships with local nurseries and garden centers is another crucial strategy for urban gardeners. These establishments are treasure troves of quality plants and expert gardening advice. Staff at these centers are typically well-educated in horticulture and can provide personalized advice specific to the local climate and urban gardening challenges. Whether dealing with pest issues, looking for the best plants for your balcony's microclimate, or needing guidance on organic gardening practices, nursery staff can offer insights based on extensive experience. Furthermore, many nurseries offer high-quality, locally sourced, or organic plants that are acclimated to the local environment, thus having a better chance of thriving in your garden. Building a rapport with your local nursery can also lead to customized service, including alerts on new arrivals and tailored recommendations that enhance your gardening success.

Community Gardens: Expanding Spaces and Fostering Community

Participation in community gardens is a unique opportunity for urban dwellers, often limited by the lack of private gardening space. These communal spaces provide the physical area necessary for gardening and foster a sense of community and collective responsibility. Engaging in a community garden allows you to cultivate a wider variety of plants, experiment with larger-scale gardening techniques, and learn from the diverse approaches of your fellow gardeners. These gardens often function as hubs of innovation and education, hosting workshops and talks that benefit the entire community. Additionally, community gardens can be instrumental in improving neighborhood green spaces, promoting biodiversity, and enhancing the overall quality of urban life. They provide a tangible connection to nature and an effective antidote to the concrete-dominated urban landscape.

Workshops and Classes: Continuous Learning and Skill Enhancement

To further enhance your gardening knowledge and skills, actively seek out workshops and classes from local botanical gardens, nurseries, or community colleges. These educational opportunities are invaluable for staying updated on the latest gardening techniques, sustainability practices, and landscape design trends. Hands-on classes offer direct experience and feedback from experts, which is crucial for mastering complex gardening skills such as pruning, grafting, or organic pest management. Workshops can also provide insights into innovative areas like vertical gardening or hydroponics, which are ideal for urban environments. Investing time in these learning opportunities enriches your practical skills and keeps you engaged and inspired in your gardening practice.

By integrating these local resources and communities into your gardening practice, you gain access to knowledge and support and contribute to a sustainable and vibrant local gardening culture. The collective benefits of these engagements can dramatically propel your gardening success, turning the challenges of urban gardening into rewarding opportunities for growth and connection.

As we conclude this exploration of essential tools and resources, the journey of a gardener is one of continuous learning and adaptation. The tools, knowledge, and networks we have discussed form the foundation of a thriving garden, supporting your growth as much as they do for your plants. The next chapter will delve into crafting your own garden accessories, further personalizing your gardening space and enhancing its functionality and aesthetic appeal. This progression from foundational knowledge to creative expression represents a holistic approach to urban gardening, ensuring that your practice is as rewarding as it is productive.

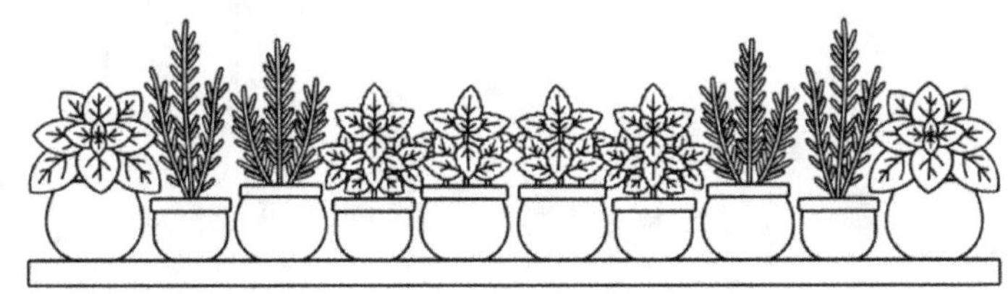

Key Chapter 9 Takeaways:

- Start with a small, intentional toolkit (pruners, watering can, soil scoop) and maintain tools through regular cleaning, sharpening, and dry storage.

- Choose ergonomic tools and smart storage solutions to reduce strain and keep gardening accessible in limited spaces.

- Use books and guides to build foundational knowledge, explore specialized topics, and troubleshoot common container-gardening problems.

- Leverage apps, websites, and plant databases to identify plants, manage watering, diagnose issues, and plan layouts with confidence.

- Strengthen your gardening success by connecting with local nurseries, clubs, community gardens, and workshops for region-specific advice and community support.

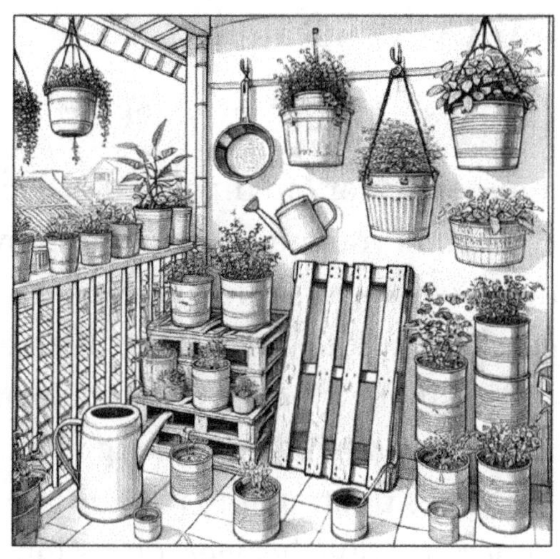

Chapter 10: Crafting Your Own Garden Accessories

Creating your own garden containers is not merely about cultivating plants; it is about shaping your immediate environment to reflect your taste and style. In urban landscapes, crafting your own containers provides a dual advantage: customization to maximize spatial efficiency and the satisfaction of enhancing your living space with a personal touch. This chapter explores foundational skills and creative insights necessary for building garden containers from scratch, transforming ordinary materials into extraordinary homes for your plants.

Building Your Own Containers

Materials and Tools: Crafting from the Ground Up

The choice of materials for building garden containers is as varied as the plants you might choose to grow within them. Traditional wood, versatile concrete, and innovative recycled materials each offer distinct advantages and aesthetic vibes. Wood stands out for its natural beauty and breathability, making it ideal for most plants, but it requires treatment to prevent rot and pest infestation. Concrete, while heavier, offers longevity and a modern look but can affect soil pH, so it may need sealing. Recycled materials, such as old barrels, tires, or kitchen containers, highlight your commitment to sustainability and can be conversation starters.

The tools required for these projects are often already present in a typical urban household or can be acquired without significant expense. A basic toolkit should include a saw for wood cutting, a drill for making drainage holes, a mixing tool for concrete, and safety gear such as gloves and goggles. Each material demands specific handling techniques: for instance, cutting wood requires precision to ensure smooth, straight edges, while mixing concrete requires careful attention to achieve the right consistency for moldability and strength.

Design Plans: Tailoring to Your Space

Designing your containers involves more than aesthetic considerations since each space is unique unto itself. Thoughtful design requires planning to ensure containers fit your available space and suit the needs of your plants. Start with measurements of your gardening area and decide on the dimensions of your containers accordingly. Consider the growth habits of the plants you wish to house. Some might need deeper containers for root development, while others might sprawl and require wider ones.

A simple online search will offer ideas for design plans and tutorials and help you visualize and execute various container styles. You will find simple box shapes ideal for beginners to more complex tiered designs that can accommodate multiple plants in a small footprint. Plans and examples can include detailed dimensions, assembly instructions, and suggested materials, providing a comprehensive guide from start to finish.

Customization Tips: Adding a Personal Touch

Once the functional aspects are addressed, customization brings your personal style into play. Painting your wooden containers can align with your patio's color scheme while embedding tiles or mosaics can turn concrete planters into art pieces. Techniques such as stenciling or decoupage allow you to personalize your containers further, making each a reflection of your personal taste.

Additionally, consider integrating functional yet decorative elements such as trellises for climbing plants or wheels for easy mobility. These adaptations enhance the utility of your containers and contribute to the overall aesthetics of your garden setup.

Safety Considerations: Ensuring Longevity and Integrity

Safety in container construction is paramount, not just for the container's longevity but also for the health of your plants and personal safety during the building process. Proper drainage is critical to prevent waterlogging and ensure plant health, requiring precise drilling of holes at the bottom of containers. Using non-toxic, water-resistant treatments for wooden containers will protect against rot without harming your plants.

Weight considerations are crucial, especially in balcony gardens, to ensure your space can structurally support your garden. Heavier materials like concrete may require reinforcement of the space or lighter alternatives. Always test the location with the weight of the container plus soil and plants to ensure stability and safety.

By embracing the DIY spirit in crafting your garden containers, you tailor your gardening space to your needs and imbue it with a sense of personal achievement and style. This chapter introduces you to the knowledge and skills to transform basic materials into functional and aesthetic plant homes, enhancing your urban garden's utility and beauty. This creation process is not just about building containers but about constructing a living space that resonates with personal creativity and ecological consciousness.

Creating Garden Markers and Labels

In the dynamic world of urban gardening, the role of garden markers and labels transcends mere identification; these elements serve as crucial navigational tools that enhance your garden's functionality and aesthetic appeal. Not only do they help distinguish between similar-looking plants, but they also provide an at-a-glance reference for plant care and tracking developmental stages.

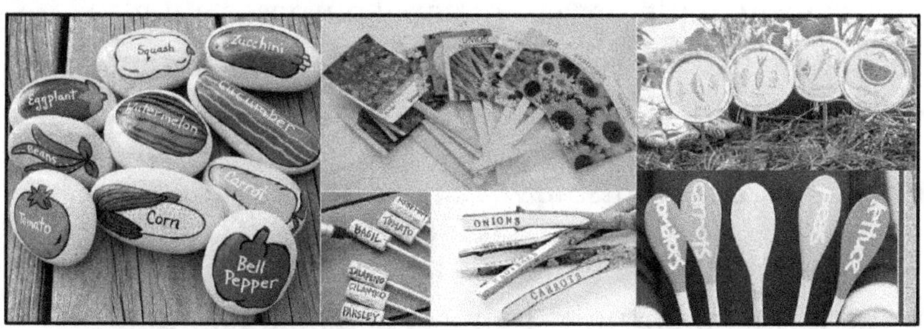

Examples of various DIY garden markers and labels

Materials: Selecting the Foundation for Your Garden Markers

The choice of material for your garden markers depends largely on the style of your garden, the durability required, and the resources available. Painted stones, for example, offer a rustic, charming option that integrates seamlessly into natural garden settings. These stones can be sourced from your local environment or purchased from garden centers, and with waterproof paint, they become decorative and weather-resistant labels. Wooden spoons, another eco-friendly option, can be repurposed from old kitchen sets or thrift store finds. They provide a flat, easily paintable surface that stands out against the greenery. For a more modern and sustainable approach, recycled plastics, cut from bottles or containers, offer a waterproof and durable marking solution. These materials not only serve functional purposes but also contribute to the aesthetic and environmental ethos of urban gardening.

Creative Ideas: Infusing Artistry into Functionality

Transforming these materials into garden markers presents an opportunity to inject personal flair and creativity into your urban garden. For painted stones, consider using vibrant colors and detailed designs that reflect the characteristics of the plant, such as leaf patterns or fruit shapes. This beautifies the garden and makes plant identification an intuitive visual experience.

Wooden spoons can be burned using a wood burning tool to create elegant, rustic labels that withstand weather elements better than paint. For recycled plastic, use permanent markers to add artistic illustrations or stenciled letters that can be customized in various fonts and sizes, aligning with the modern, minimalist aesthetic prevalent in urban settings.

Organization Tips: Enhancing Garden Management

Beyond aesthetics, the practical function of garden markers in managing your plant care regime is invaluable. Accurate labeling assists in tracking the growth progress, understanding seasonal changes, and maintaining timely care schedules. It prevents confusion, especially in gardens with various plants, and simplifies maintenance routines. Implementing a system that includes the plant name, sowing date, and specific care instructions directly on the marker can save time and enhance the efficiency of your gardening practices. For those managing more extensive or complex gardens, consider creating a coded system corresponding to detailed notes in a gardening journal, allowing for more comprehensive tracking and historical data accumulation.

By integrating these customized garden markers into your urban gardening strategy, you will streamline your gardening operations and elevate your space's visual and functional appeal. This approach reflects a commitment to organization and care and showcases a fusion of utility and personal artistic expression, making urban gardening a truly enriching activity.

Small-Scale Water Features for Container Gardens

Creating a water feature for your urban garden transforms an ordinary container garden into an enchanting oasis that captivates the senses and offers environmental benefits. Simple, small-scale water features such as tabletop fountains and bubbling water pots can be easily constructed, providing a dynamic element to your garden setting. For those with limited space, a tabletop fountain offers a compact solution that can be placed on a balcony table or a window ledge, effectively enhancing the ambiance with the soothing sound of trickling water. Alternatively, bubbling water pots, crafted using submersible pumps in any watertight container, create a gentle bubbling effect that adds a serene audiovisual experience to your garden.

Select a small, waterproof basin as the base to begin constructing a tabletop fountain. This could be a ceramic bowl or a small decorative pot. A submersible pump, easily available at garden centers or online, is placed at the bottom of this basin. The pump should be covered with decorative stones or small pebbles to create a natural look and to hide the mechanical parts. Water is added to the container, ensuring the pump is fully submerged. The pump circulates the water, creating a continuous flow from the stone-covered top, providing the delightful sound of falling water. The setup is similar for those opting for a bubbling water pot, but instead of directing the water to flow over the top, the pump settings can be adjusted to create a bubbling effect right at the water's surface. A quick internet search will yield a variety of other options that will fit the style of your garden.

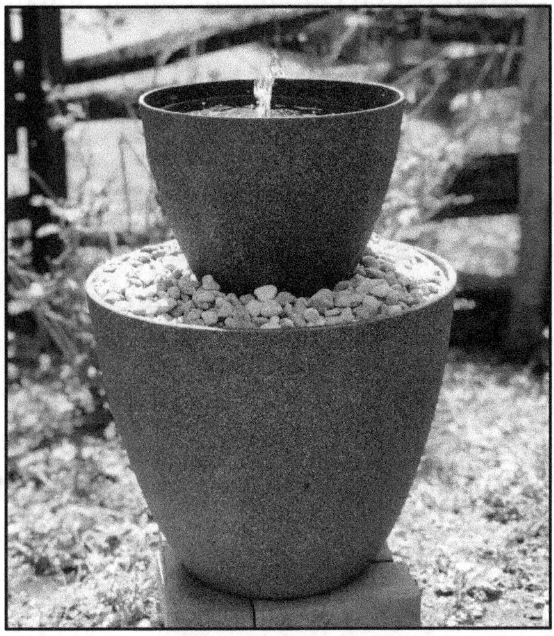

Example of a small-space-friendly water feature

The benefits of incorporating such water features into your container garden are manifold. Aesthetically, they provide a focal point that draws the eye, adding movement and sound to make even the smallest spaces feel more expansive and alive. Environmentally, water features contribute significantly to the local microclimate by adding humidity to the air, which can be particularly beneficial in urban areas prone to dry conditions. This increase in humidity is welcomed by many plants, potentially improving their health and growth. Furthermore, the sound of water is a natural attractant for wildlife, encouraging birds and beneficial insects to visit your garden, which can aid in pollination and natural pest control.

Maintaining these water features ensures their effectiveness and longevity. Regular cleaning is essential to prevent the buildup of algae and debris, which could clog the pump and interrupt the water flow. It is advisable to clean the pump and change the water bi-weekly, using a brush to scrub the interior surfaces of the basin or pot to keep it free from algae. In the colder months, if temperatures drop below freezing, it's important to either remove the pump and store it indoors or ensure that the water feature is completely drained to prevent damage from freezing.

Integrating water features with container plants requires thoughtful placement and selection of accompanying flora. Positioning a small water feature near plants that thrive in humid conditions, such as ferns or hostas, can create a micro-habitat that maximizes growth and vitality. Additionally, consider the aesthetics of how the water feature complements the plant arrangement. For example, a bubbling pot surrounded by low-growing, lush greenery can mimic the appearance of a natural spring, while a tabletop fountain placed amongst tall, flowering plants can mimic a rainforest environment, making your garden not only a place of growth but also a sanctuary of peace and natural beauty.

DIY Pest Deterrents and Attractants

To maintain a healthy urban garden, managing pests without resorting to harsh chemicals is both an art and a science. Urban gardeners often face unique challenges due to the proximity of their plants to living spaces and the ecological sensibilities accompanying urban life. This subchapter explores effective, environmentally friendly methods for deterring pests and attracting beneficial insects, utilizing common household ingredients and simple DIY projects. These strategies enhance the health and productivity of your garden and align with sustainable gardening practices, crucial in urban settings.

Natural Repellents: Harnessing the Power of Nature

Creating natural pest repellents is a practical approach to garden maintenance that minimizes harm to the environment and your plants. Common kitchen ingredients such as garlic, chili, and various herbs possess properties that can deter pests naturally. A simple yet effective repellent can be made by blending garlic cloves and hot peppers with a small amount of water, creating a potent mixture that can be diluted and sprayed directly onto plant leaves. This mixture is a strong deterrent against many pests, including aphids and beetles, due to the natural compounds in garlic and chili that pests find unpalatable. Learn more about making natural pest repellents in Appendix 7 on page 255.

Herbs like basil, lavender, and lemongrass can be planted strategically around your garden to repel insects naturally. These herbs contain essential oils that many pests dislike, and their presence can help to create a pest-resistant barrier around more sensitive plants. Planting these herbs in containers around your garden not only adds to the diversity and beauty of your space but also plays a crucial role in your integrated pest management strategy.

Attracting Beneficial Insects: Cultivating Biological Defenders

Attracting beneficial insects such as ladybugs, bees, and lacewings is another cornerstone of natural pest control. These insects are natural predators of many common garden pests and play a pivotal role in maintaining the ecological balance within your garden. Creating insect hotels is a simple DIY project that can enhance the population of beneficial insects in your area. Using materials such as bamboo tubes, straw, and untreated wood, you can construct a shelter that provides these creatures with the nooks and crannies they need for nesting and hibernating.

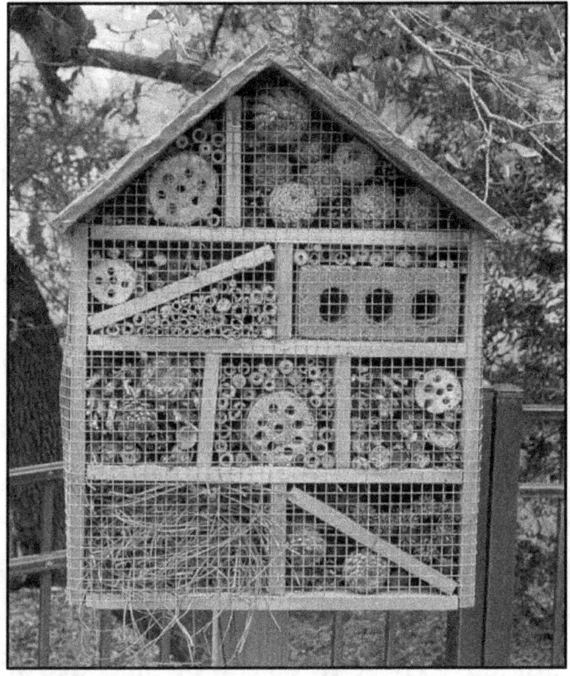

Example of a DIY insect hotel

In addition to building insect hotels, planting insectary flowers like marigolds, sunflowers, and cosmos can attract beneficial insects. These flowers provide nectar and pollen that are essential for the survival of these insects, encouraging them to take up residence in your garden. As a result, they help in controlling pest populations naturally, reducing the need for manual intervention.

Barriers and Traps: Fortifying Your Garden Defenses

Physical barriers and traps are effective tools in the gardener's arsenal for preventing pests from reaching plant foliage. Copper tape can be applied around the rims of pots or beds to deter slugs and snails. Their mucous membranes react with the copper, causing them to receive a mild electric shock upon contact. This method is particularly useful in container gardens, where each plant can be individually protected.

Homemade sticky traps can also be crafted to catch flying insects such as whiteflies and fungus gnats. Bright colors like yellow or blue, which attract these pests, can be used to coat plastic or cardboard with a sticky substance such as petroleum jelly. These traps can be placed around the garden, especially near plants prone to these pests. Regularly monitoring and replacing these traps can provide you with insight into pest populations, allowing for timely interventions.

Maintenance and Monitoring: Keeping a Vigilant Eye

The effectiveness of DIY pest control solutions hinges on consistent maintenance and vigilant monitoring. Regular checks of your garden for signs of pest activity are crucial in detecting potential issues before they escalate. This includes examining the undersides of leaves, checking for plant damage, and assessing the health of your traps and barriers. Keeping a garden journal can help track these observations, allowing you to identify patterns or recurring problems that can inform your future pest management strategies.

Moreover, maintaining the cleanliness and order of your garden by removing debris and dead plants reduces the chances of pests finding a comfortable habitat to thrive. Ensuring that your DIY deterrents and attractants are well-maintained and strategically placed can significantly affect their effectiveness. This proactive approach keeps your garden healthy and aligns with the principles of sustainable urban gardening by fostering a natural balance that supports plant health and local ecosystems.

Making Your Own Plant Supports

In the dynamic and often spatially constrained world of urban gardening, providing adequate support for your plants is not merely a practical necessity but also an opportunity to enhance your garden's structural and visual appeal. As various plants, particularly climbers and tall species, reach towards the sunlight, they require support systems that are both functional and harmonious with the garden's overall design. This section explores the creation of homemade plant supports, such as trellises, stakes, and cages, which you can construct using easily accessible materials, offering a perfect blend of utility and aesthetic charm.

Support Types: Diverse Options for Plant Stability

The choice of support type largely depends on the specific needs of your plants and your personal design preferences. Trellises are ideal for climbing plants like ivy, cucumbers, and climbing roses, providing a vertical plane that supports growth and contributes to air circulation and sun exposure, which is essential for plant health. Stakes offer a straightforward solution for upright growth support, suitable for plants like tomatoes and young trees that might otherwise succumb to the weight of their fruit or wind. Cages, particularly useful for bushy plants such as peonies and some types of vegetables like peppers, help maintain plant structure and protect the plant from external damage.

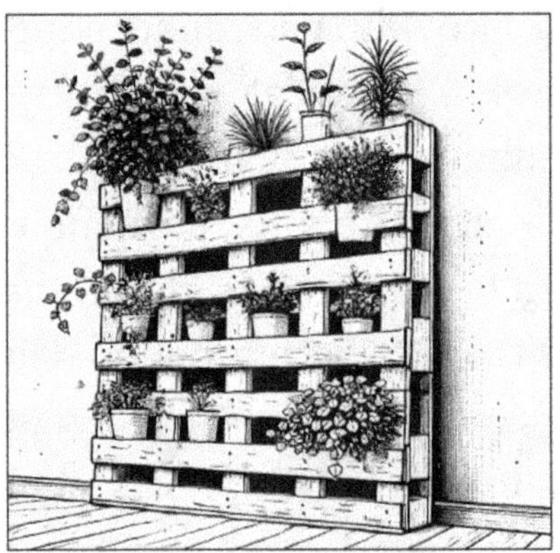

Constructing these supports at home allows customization to fit specific garden layouts and aesthetic visions. For instance, a trellis can be tailored in size and shape, incorporating curves or angles that complement the architectural elements of your living space. A cage can be crafted to accommodate the anticipated size of a mature plant, ensuring it is both supportive and unobtrusive.

Materials: Selecting Sustainable and Effective Options

The choice of materials for constructing plant supports should reflect considerations of durability, environmental impact, and visual impact. Upcycled materials, such as bamboo poles, old wooden planks, or even metal rods from discarded furniture, can be repurposed to create sturdy and eco-friendly supports. Bamboo, in particular, is highly recommended due to its strength, flexibility, and sustainability, making it ideal for both stakes and trellises. Metal rods or wire can be shaped into cages or intricate trellis designs, offering functionality combined with industrial chic aesthetics that can contrast beautifully with the organic forms of plant life.

When selecting materials, consider the environmental conditions they will be exposed to. Wood, while visually appealing and easy to work with, may require treatment with eco-friendly preservatives to prevent rot in damp climates. Metals should be rust-proofed to maintain their structural integrity and appearance. Each material choice carries implications for the longevity and maintenance needs of the plant supports and, as such, should align with the practical realities of your urban garden environment.

Construction Tips: Building for Durability and Effectiveness

Constructing plant supports requires a blend of craftsmanship and understanding plant behavior. When building a trellis, ensure that the spacing between the slats or mesh is appropriate for the type of plant it is intended to support. Climbers, for instance, need closely spaced supports to latch onto as they grow, whereas broader-spaced designs may suit ornamental plants that require more visual exposure. Secure joints and a stable base are crucial to prevent collapse under the weight of mature plants. Techniques such as interlocking joints for wooden frames or welded connections for metal supports can enhance the durability and safety of your constructions.

For stakes, pointed ends can be created for easier insertion into the soil, reducing disturbance to the plant roots. If wood is chosen as the material, a coating of natural wax or oil can help preserve it. Cages require careful consideration of diameter and height to accommodate growth without constriction, with modular designs allowing for adjustments as plants mature.

Aesthetic Integration: Harmonizing Function and Style

Integrating plant supports into your garden's design aesthetic involves more than selecting materials that match your décor. It includes considering the form and function of the supports as integral components of the garden's visual and spatial composition. Trellises can be used as plant supports and screens to delineate spaces within your garden or hide less attractive areas. Stakes and cages can be painted or decorated as visual highlights rather than just functional elements.

Incorporating climbing plants on trellises or arranging containers with stakes in a visually pleasing pattern can transform these supports into focal points of your garden. Integrating these elements should feel intentional and thoughtful, enhancing the overall cohesiveness of your urban gardening space and turning functional necessities into key components of your garden's charm and character.

Upcycling Ideas for Garden Art

The realm of upcycling in garden art is a testament to the adage that one person's trash is another's treasure. Viewing everyday objects through the lens of creativity allows for transforming mundane items into unique, eco-friendly pieces that enhance the aesthetic of any urban garden. This approach elevates your space's visual appeal and underscores a commitment to environmental stewardship, turning waste reduction into an art form.

Inspiration for Upcycling: Seeing the Artistic in the Ordinary

Inspiration for your upcycling projects can be found in the most ordinary and unexpected places. Old kitchen items, discarded furniture, or broken ceramics can all be given new life as garden art. The process begins with viewing these items not as waste but as potential treasures. For example, consider how an old car tire can be repurposed into a vibrant garden planter or how a collection of mismatched teacups can become a charming bird feeder. Start by exploring your home or local thrift shops and salvage yards in places where these items are often abundant and inexpensive. By incorporating these reclaimed items into your garden, you create a unique space and contribute to a cycle of renewal and sustainability.

Project Ideas: Crafting Beauty from Discards

Turning these found objects into garden art can be both fun and fulfilling. Consider the tire planter project: tires can be painted in bright, durable outdoor paint and filled with soil and plants, creating a striking, whimsical flower display. Similarly, old glass bottles can be transformed into wind chimes or garden edging, catching the light and adding a splash of color and sound to your garden. Another creative project involves using old wooden spoons as plant markers, painted or carved with the names of the plants they signify. These projects personalize your garden space and act as conversation starters, showcasing your creativity and environmental awareness.

Creative Process: Cultivating Your Artistic Garden Vision

The creative process in upcycling for garden art involves several stages, beginning with collecting and selecting materials. This is followed by envisioning the potential transformations these items can undergo. Sketching your ideas can be a helpful way to visualize the end products and plan the necessary steps to achieve them. This process might involve painting, cutting, assembling, or other modifications, depending on the nature of the project. It's important to allow yourself the freedom to experiment and embrace imperfections. Often, the quirks and unexpected outcomes can enhance the charm of upcycled art.

During this creative journey, consider the functional aspects of your artistic creations. For instance, ensure that any containers or planters provide adequate drainage for plants and that any decorative items added to the garden are weather-resistant or appropriately protected. Engaging in this creative process not only refines your crafting skills but also deepens your connection to your garden as a dynamic canvas for your artistic expression.

Environmental Impact: Advocating for Sustainability through Art

The environmental impact of upcycling in garden art extends beyond waste reduction. Repurposing items reduces the demand for new products and the resources and energy required to produce them. This practice sets a valuable example of environmental responsibility, inspiring others to consider sustainability in their gardening and lifestyle choices. Moreover, upcycled garden art often uses locally sourced materials, further reducing the carbon footprint associated with transporting goods.

Incorporating upcycled art into your garden transforms it into a showcase of sustainable practices, blending aesthetics with environmental ethics. This approach beautifies your space and contributes to a larger movement towards ecological consciousness and resourcefulness, making each upcycled piece a testament to the possibilities inherent in reimagining and repurposing.

As this chapter closes, we reflect on the transformative power of upcycling in converting everyday objects into valuable garden art. This practice beautifies your urban garden space while underscoring the importance of sustainability. It reveals the hidden potential in what many would consider waste, turning it into something both beautiful and useful.

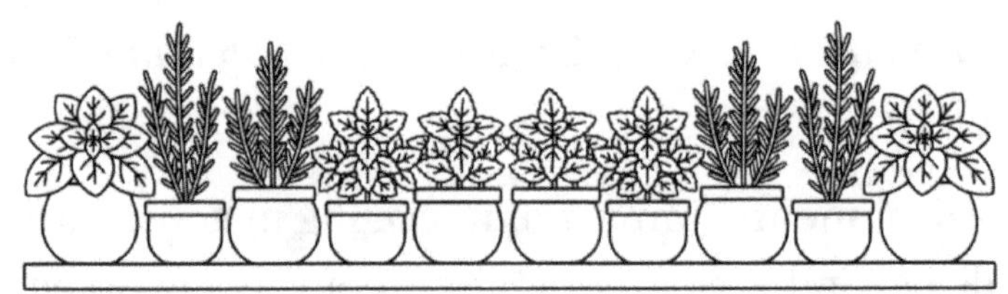

Key Chapter 10 Takeaways:

- Build containers with material choice, plant needs, drainage, space constraints, and balcony weight limits in mind

- Use customization (paint, mosaic, wheels, trellises) to make containers functional and personal.

- Create garden markers that do more than label: include plant name + date + care notes to support consistent management.

- Add a small water feature to boost ambience, humidity, and wildlife visits, and keep it working with simple cleaning routines.

- Use DIY pest strategies that combine repellents + beneficial insect support + barriers + monitoring for long-term balance.

- Make plant supports from accessible materials and treat them as part of your garden design, not an afterthought.

- Upcycle everyday objects into garden art to reduce waste and create a unique, story-filled container garden space.

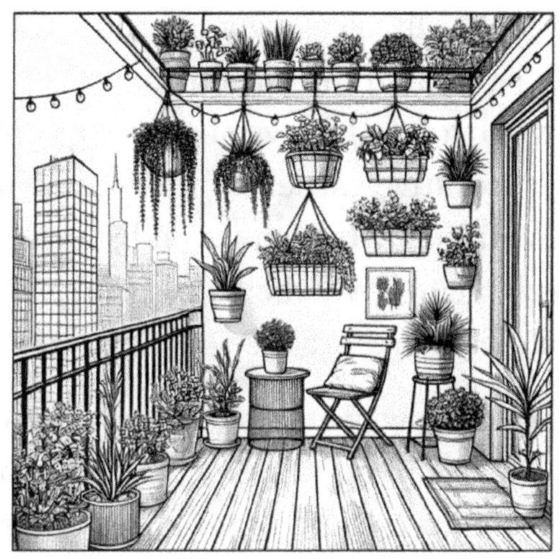

Conclusion

As we reach the conclusion of this enriching and exciting journey through *"CONTAINER GARDENING for BEGINNERS"* let us take a moment to reflect on the transformative experience that container gardening offers. We have explored how even the most compact urban spaces can be magically turned into lush, thriving gardens. This book has equipped you with the knowledge and confidence to bring the vibrancy of nature into your home, demonstrating that the size of your space need not limit the scope of your green aspirations.

Throughout this guide, we delved into the essentials of container gardening, from selecting the right containers and understanding soil composition to mastering the art of watering and fertilization. We navigated through designing aesthetically pleasing and productive spaces, embraced the rhythm of the seasons to maximize garden vitality, and discovered the joys of growing edible plants and creating decorative gardens. Innovative gardening techniques, including hydroponics and smart gardening solutions, were uncovered, offering advanced methods to enhance your gardening practice.

One of the core messages of this book has been the accessibility of gardening. You do not need vast tracts of land or years of horticultural experience to start. Container gardening opens up a world where anyone can participate in the act of growing, bringing simplicity and joy into the bustling life of urban dwellers. It dispels the myth that gardening is beyond the reach of those without gardens grounded in the earth.

We have also emphasized sustainability and wellness, integrating themes like upcycling and organic gardening. These practices respect our planet and enrich our lives, making gardening a deeply therapeutic activity that can improve mental and physical health. The DIY projects we explored are more than just functional; they are a creative expression that enhances the personal connection to your garden.

I encourage you to continue expanding your gardening knowledge and skills. Engage with local gardening communities and tap into online resources and forums. These platforms are invaluable for sharing insights and experiences that can refine your gardening techniques. Remember, the learning never stops, and every season brings new lessons and opportunities.

Gardening is inherently personal and creative. I urge you to experiment with different plant choices, designs, and projects that reflect your unique style and preferences. Partner with local nurseries or garden stores to select the best plants and varieties for your region, ensuring your garden is beautiful and thriving.

With the insights and techniques garnered from this book, I challenge you to either embark on your gardening journey or elevate your existing garden to new heights. Start small, think big, and grow your garden with intention and creativity.

Lastly, I invite you to share your gardening stories. Whether they are of success, challenge, or continuous learning, your stories can inspire and encourage a community of like-minded individuals who are also on their own gardening adventures. By sharing, we foster a collective spirit of support and enrichment.

In conclusion, remember that gardening reconnects us with the natural world even on the smallest balcony or windowsill. It transforms our living spaces, brings unparalleled beauty into our daily lives, and offers a sustainable path to enhancing our well-being. Continue to nurture your garden, which will nurture you back in ways you never imagined. Here's to the magic that gardening brings into our lives. May it flourish in your hands.

Your feedback is greatly appreciated!

Your feedback, support, and reviews make it possible for us to create high-quality books and serve more people.

It only takes 60 seconds to leave an honest review. Share your feedback and thoughts so others can see the quality of this book.

Find the location where you purchased the book and leave a review. Select a rating and write a couple of sentences.

That's it! Thank you so much for your support.

Review this product

Share your thoughts with other customers

Write a customer review

Appendix 1 - 8

Appendix 1

Rotation of plants

Year 1:

Leafy Greens	Lettuce Spinach Swiss chard	Leafy greens generally have shallow roots and use less nitrogen. Starting with these plants prepares the soil without exhausting it.

Year 2:

Fruiting Vegetables	Tomatoes Peppers Eggplants	These plants are heavy feeders, especially of nutrients like nitrogen, which would be conserved in the soil from the previous year's lighter-feeding leafy greens.

Year 3:

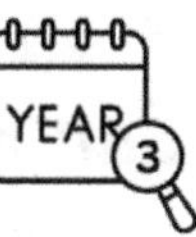

Root Vegetables	Carrots Radishes Beets	Root vegetables can benefit from the loosened soil left by the deep roots of tomatoes and peppers. They also help break up the soil, improving its structure.

Year 4:

Legumes	Beans Peas	Legumes fix nitrogen back into the soil, replenishing it after the nutrients have been significantly used up by the previous crops. This sets the stage well for leafy greens again in the next rotation cycle.

Additional Rotation Tips:

Herbs	Can generally be rotated in any of these years as most herbs are not heavy feeders. However, it's best to avoid planting herbs that might interfere with the soil's balance, such as mint, which can be invasive even in containers.
Onions and Garlic	These can be used in the year before planting fruiting vegetables as they can help deter some pests and diseases naturally

Appendix 2

Companion Planting: Plant these together.

Vegetables

 Tomatoes and Basil	Basil helps repel flies and mosquitoes, and some gardeners believe it can improve the flavor of tomatoes.
Lettuce and Chives or Garlic	Chives and garlic deter aphids, which are common pests on lettuce.

Carrots and Rosemary	Rosemary repels carrot flies and bean beetles, making it a good companion for carrots and beans.
Peppers and Basil	Basil can help repel thrips, flies and mosquitoes, potentially improving the growth and flavor of peppers.
Cucumbers and Nasturtiums	Nasturtiums are known to repel cucumber beetles and can act as a trap crop, luring pests away from cucumbers.
Spinach and Strawberries	Growing spinach and strawberries together utilizes vertical space, as spinach can grow in the shade provided by strawberry plants.
Eggplant and Thyme	Thyme repels the eggplant flea beetle, a common pest for eggplants.
Sage and Rosemary	Both herbs thrive in similar dry conditions and can help deter cabbage moths and carrot flies.

**Oregano and Peppers**	Oregano acts as a general pest repellent, making it beneficial near many vegetables.
Cilantro and Spinach	Cilantro helps repel pests from spinach, and both can tolerate cooler temperatures.
Parsley and Tomato	Parsley can enhance the growth and flavor of tomatoes while also attracting beneficial insects.

Flowers

Marigolds and Almost Anything	Marigolds are fantastic companions for many plants. They repel pests like nematodes and beetles and can be particularly effective when grown with tomatoes or peppers.
Lavender and Roses	Lavender can help deter aphids and other pests from roses. It also attracts pollinators and adds fragrance and contrast to the visual appeal.

Geraniums and Peppers or Cabbage	Geraniums can repel cabbage worms and Japanese beetles, making them good companions for cabbage, broccoli, and peppers.
Petunias and Beans	Petunias repel bean beetles and can add a splash of color to your container garden while protecting bean plants.
Zinnias and Cauliflower	Zinnias can attract ladybugs and other predators that help control pests attacking cauliflower.
Calendula and Almost Any Vegetable	Known as the "pot marigold," calendula is great at attracting beneficial insects that prey on pests troubling nearby vegetables.
Snapdragons and Spinach	Snapdragons attract bumblebees which are effective pollinators and can help increase spinach yield.

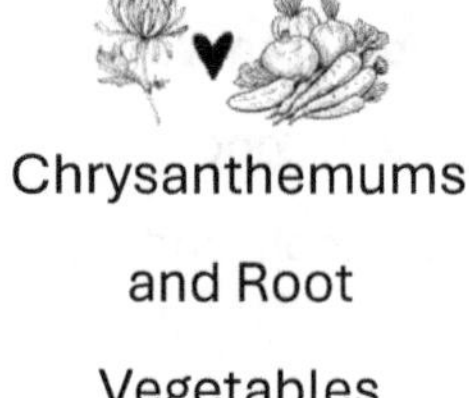 Chrysanthemums and Root Vegetables	Chrysanthemums contain a natural insecticide called pyrethrin, which helps protect root vegetables like carrots and radishes from soil-borne pests.

Appendix 3

Do not plant together

Herbs and Vegetables 

Beans and Onions (including garlic, leeks, and shallots)	Onions and other alliums can stunt the growth of beans by inhibiting their ability to absorb nitrogen, a crucial nutrient for beans.
Carrots and Dill	Dill can attract carrot root flies, which will damage the carrots. Dill may inhibit carrot growth when planted too close.

Cucumbers and Aromatic Herbs (like sage or basil)	Strong-smelling herbs can stunt the growth of cucumbers by releasing chemicals that interfere with cucumber development.
Tomatoes and Potatoes	Both being members of the nightshade family, they can easily transmit blight to each other, a disease that can devastate both crops.
Asparagus and Garlic	Garlic can stunt the growth of asparagus. Similarly, onions and other alliums have a negative impact on asparagus.
Peppers and Beans	Beans fix nitrogen in the soil, which peppers do not like in high amounts. They are both prone to the same diseases, which can spread easily if they are planted together.
Kale and Tomatoes	Tomatoes can spread fungal diseases to kale, impacting its growth and health.
Peas and Onions	Onions can inhibit the growth of peas by interfering with nitrogen absorption.

<table>
<tr>
<td>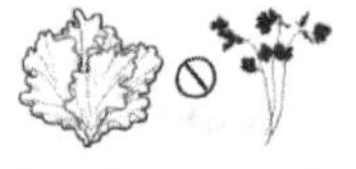
Lettuce and
Parsley</td>
<td>Parsley can overtake the space and shade out the lettuce, which needs plenty of light to grow well.</td>
</tr>
</table>

Flowers

<table>
<tr>
<td>Sunflowers and
Pot Marigolds
(Calendula)</td>
<td>Sunflowers have large root systems that can strangle the roots of smaller plants like calendula, depriving them of essential nutrients and water.</td>
</tr>
<tr>
<td>Daffodils and
Tulips</td>
<td>Daffodils secrete a substance that can inhibit the growth of tulips when planted in close proximity, potentially causing poor growth or bulb damage.</td>
</tr>
<tr>
<td>Roses and
Clematis</td>
<td>While often planted together in the ground, in containers, the heavy feeding nature of roses can compete too aggressively with clematis, leading to nutrient deprivation for the clematis.</td>
</tr>
</table>

Lavender and Begonias	Lavender prefers dry conditions with well-draining soil, while begonias thrive in more moist environments, making their watering needs incompatible.
Lilies and Gladiolus	Both plants are heavy feeders and compete for the same nutrients, which can lead to stunted growth when confined in a container.
Asters and Impatiens	Asters require well-draining soil conditions, whereas impatiens prefer consistently moist soil, making their water needs incompatible.
Zinnias and Cosmos	Both zinnias and cosmos are susceptible to powdery mildew, planting them together in a confined space can increase the likelihood of disease transmission.

Appendix 4

Pollinator plants

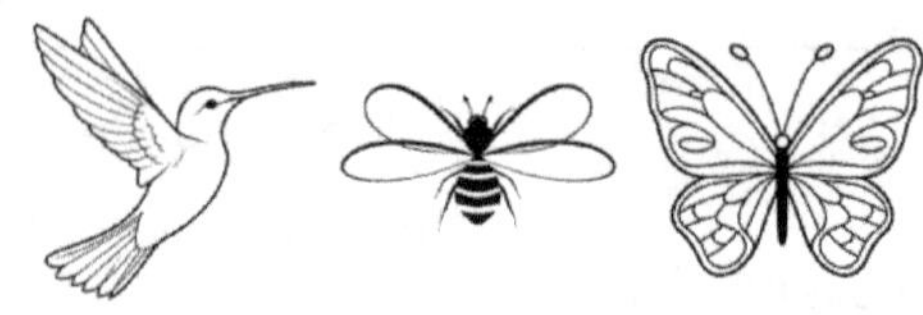

Lavender	Lavender's rich nectar attracts bees and butterflies, and its fragrant foliage can deter deer and other pests.
Marigolds	These bright flowers are excellent for attracting bees, and their strong scent can help repel unwanted insects that might harm other plants.
Zinnias	Zinnias are a favorite of butterflies and hummingbirds due to their vibrant colors and abundant nectar.
Salvia	Available in several varieties, salvias are beloved by bees and hummingbirds for their prolonged blooming period.
Cosmos	Easy to grow and with daisy-like flowers, cosmos attract bees and butterflies throughout the summer.

Geraniums	Some geraniums are especially good at attracting bees, and they are very easy to grow in containers.
Coneflower (Echinacea)	Coneflowers are known for attracting butterflies and bees, and their seeds are favored by birds in the fall and winter.
Butterfly Bush (Buddleia)	Though larger, this shrub can be grown in containers and is a magnet for butterflies.
Alyssum	Its tiny flowers are loved by small beneficial insects, including hoverflies and parasitic wasps that help control pest populations.
Fuchsia	Fuchsia's unique flowers attract hummingbirds and can be grown in hanging baskets or pots.

Appendix 5

Hydroponic Gardening

Plants Suitable for Hydroponic Gardening

Lettuce	Thrives in hydroponics due to its low nutritional requirements and rapid growth cycle.
Spinach	Adapts well to hydroponic systems, which can prevent soil-borne diseases and provide consistent water, enhancing leaf production.
Strawberries	Benefit from hydroponic systems as they receive an even, consistent supply of water and nutrients, reducing common soil-related issues and pests.
Bell Peppers	Grow well hydroponically, receiving optimal nutrients and water which can result in higher yields and faster growth compared to soil gardening.
Tomatoes	Suited to hydroponic systems due to their high water and nutrient needs, which can be more precisely managed in such setups, promoting healthier growth and productivity.

Herbs (such as basil, mint, and parsley)	These generally have shallow roots and thrive in hydroponic systems where their water and minimal nutritional needs are easily met, leading to lush growth.
Cucumbers	Excel in hydroponic systems because of their fast growth and high-water requirements, which can be efficiently met in a controlled water-based environment.
Kale	Benefits from the controlled nutrient management in hydroponic systems, which promotes faster growth and larger leaves, free from soil-borne pests.
Swiss Chard	Adapts well to hydroponics, enjoying the constant moisture and nutrients that lead to rapid and vibrant leaf production.
Bok Choy	Grows exceptionally well in hydroponic systems, which provide the consistent moisture and nutrients needed for its quick growth cycle.
Green Beans	Can be grown in hydroponic systems where they receive a steady supply of nutrients, promoting continuous growth and yield.

Radishes	Ideal for hydroponic cultivation due to their rapid growth and minimal space requirements, yielding results much faster than soil cultivation.
Chilies	Suitable for hydroponics as they require consistent conditions of warmth and nutrients which can be precisely controlled in such systems, leading to better fruit production.
Peas	They do well as the hydroponic systems allow for vertical growth setups, maximizing space and providing the necessary water and nutrients directly to the roots.
Watercress	Naturally a water-loving plant, it excels in hydroponic systems where it can receive abundant moisture, enhancing its growth and flavor.
Orchids	These can flourish in non-traditional hydroponic setups, as they naturally grow in air or on other surfaces rather than in soil, benefiting from the excellent drainage and airflow.

Plants NOT Suitable for Hydroponic Gardening

Potatoes	These root vegetables require a large amount of substrate for rooting and tuber formation, which is difficult to provide in standard hydroponic setups.
Carrots	Like other root vegetables, carrots need deep, solid media to form properly, which isn't ideally provided by typical hydroponic systems.
Zucchini and Squash	These plants are typically large and sprawling with heavy fruits that require extensive support structures when grown hydroponically, making them less suitable.
Corn	Corn grows tall and can become top-heavy, requiring substantial support and space, which is challenging to manage in hydroponic systems.
Berries (like raspberries and blackberries)	These plants generally require a large amount of space for their root systems and can be difficult to manage hydroponically due to their perennial nature and need for seasonal dormancy.

Woody Herbs (like rosemary)	These can be grown hydroponically but often do not thrive as they prefer drier conditions and can suffer from root issues in the constantly moist hydroponics environment.
Melons	While it's possible to grow melons hydroponically, their large space requirements and heavy fruiting can make them impractical and less efficient in a hydroponic setup.

Appendix 6

Common Nutrient Deficiencies and Their Solutions

Nitrogen (N) Deficiency

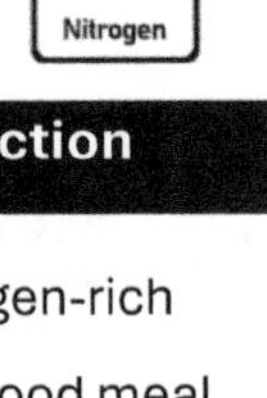

Symptoms	Identification	Correction
Yellowing of older leaves Stunted growth Pale overall plant color.	Older leaves turn pale green or yellow, starting from the tips. Plant growth is slowed.	Use a nitrogen-rich fertilizer (blood meal, fish emulsion) Maintain soil pH between 6.0-7.0 to support nitrogen uptake.

Phosphorous (P) Deficiency

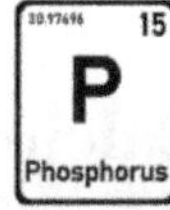

Symptoms	Identification	Correction
Dark green leaves that may turn purplish or reddish Poor root development Delayed flowering	Older leaves develop a dull green appearance followed by purple or red tones Overall plant growth and root expansion may be slow.	Apply a phosphorous-rich fertilizer (bone meal, rock phosphate) Maintain soil pH to 6.0-7.0

Potassium (K) Deficiency

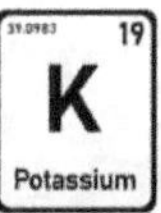

Symptoms	Identification	Correction
Yellowing or browning at leaf edges Weak stems Poor fruit and flower development	Older leaves show yellowing at the margins and tips, which may progress inward. Leaf edges may appear scorched or curled	Use potassium-rich fertilizers (potassium sulfate, kelp meal, wood ash) Maintain a soil pH of 6.0-7.0.

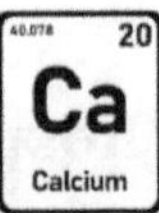

Calcium (Ca) Deficiency

Symptoms	Identification	Correction
Blossom end rot in tomatoes, peppers Tip burn in lettuce Distorted new leaves	Young leaves are distorted or hook shaped. Fruits may develop dark, sunken spots.	Apply calcium sources (lime, gypsum) Ensure consistent watering to help calcium absorption.

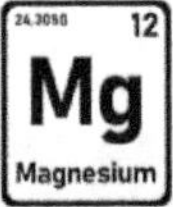

Magnesium (Mg) Deficiency

Symptoms	Identification	Correction
Yellowing leaf veins on older leaves Leaves may develop reddish or purple tones in advanced stages	Yellowing of leaf tissue between the veins while veins remain green. Symptoms progress upward if untreated.	Apply Epsom salt as a soil drench (2 Tbsp : 1 gallon water) Maintain soil pH between6.0-7.0

Iron (Fe) Deficiency 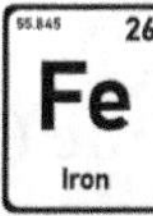

Symptoms	Identification	Correction
Yellowing between veins on new leaves	Young leaves turn yellow between the veins, while veins remain green.	Apply iron chelates or ferrous sulfate Ensure the soil pH is slightly acidic (5.5-6.5).

Manganese (Mn) Deficiency 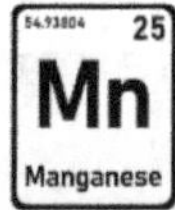

Symptoms	Identification	Correction
Yellowing between veins on younger leaves, similar to iron deficiency, but with dead spots	Young leaves show yellowing between veins, sometimes accompanied by brown spots.	Use manganese sulfate or manganese chelates Maintain a slightly acidic soil pH (5.5-6.5).

Zinc (Zn) Deficiency

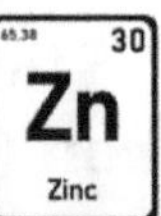

Symptoms	Identification	Correction
Stunted growth Small leaves Yellowing between veins on older leaves	Leaves are smaller than usual Leaves may yellow, accompanied by bronzing.	Apply zinc sulfate or zinc chelates Maintain a soil pH of 5.5-7.0.

General Tips for Correcting Nutrient Deficiencies

Soil Testing	Conduct a soil test to diagnose deficiencies and adjust nutrient levels accordingly.
Balanced Fertilizers	Use a balanced, complete fertilizer to prevent multiple nutrient deficiencies.
Organic Matter	Incorporate compost or well-rotted manure to improve nutrient availability and soil structure
pH Management	Maintain proper soil pH to ensure optimal nutrient uptake. Most nutrients are best available in a pH range of 6-7.
Consistent Watering	Ensure consistent watering practices, as fluctuations can affect nutrient uptake.

Appendix 7

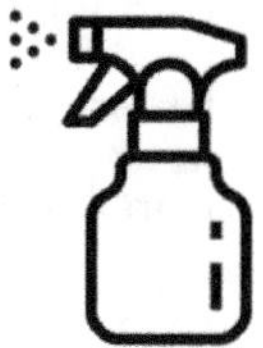

DIY Natural Pest Repellents

Neem Oil Spray

1 teaspoon neem oil 1/2 teaspoon mild liquid soap (castile soap works well) 1 quart (1 liter) water	Mix neem oil and liquid soap in a spray bottle. Add water and shake well to combine.	Effective against aphids, spider mites, whiteflies, and fungal diseases. Spray on plants every 7-14 days as a preventative measure or directly on pests for treatment.

Garlic Spray

1 garlic bulb 4 cups (1 liter) water 1 teaspoon mild liquid soap	Blend the garlic bulb with 2 cups (500 ml) water and let it steep overnight. Strain the mixture and add liquid soap.	Repels aphids, ants, and beetles. Spray on plants once a week or after rain. *(continued)*

(Garlic Spray continued)	Pour into a spray bottle and dilute with an additional 2 cups (500 ml) of water.	

Soap Spray

2 Tablespoons mild liquid soap 1 quart (1 liter) water	Mix soap and water in a spray bottle. Shake well to combine.	Effective against soft-bodied insects like aphids, whiteflies, and spider mites. Spray directly on pests every 4-7 days.

Baking Soda Spray

1 Tablespoon Baking Soda 1 teaspoon mild liquid soap 1 gallon (4 liters) water	Mix baking soda and liquid soap in a gallon of water. Pour into spray bottle.	Prevents and treats fungal diseases like powdery mildew. Spray on plants every 7-14 days.

Eucalyptus Spray

10 drops eucalyptus essential oil 1 quart (1 liter) water	Add eucalyptus oil to water in a spray bottle. Shake well to combine.	Repels mosquitoes, flies, and other flying insects. Spray on plants as needed.

Citrus Oil Spray

10 drops citrus essential oil (lemon, orange, or lime) 1 quart (1 liter) water	Mix citrus oil with water in a spray bottle. Shake well to combine.	Deters aphids, ants, and gnats. Spray on plants as needed.

Herbal Oil Spray

1 Tablespoon dried basil, mint, or rosemary 1 quart (1 liter) water	Boil water and pour over dried herbs. Let steep until cool, then strain.	Repels a variety of insects including aphids, mites, and whiteflies. *(continued)*

	Pour into a spray bottle.	Spray on plants every 7-14 days.
(Herbal Oil Spray continued)		

Appendix 8

Further Resources

Books

Book	Author	Details
"The Vegetable Gardener's Container Bible"	Edward C. Smith	demystifies growing vegetables in containers
"Container Gardening Complete"	Jessica Walliser	how-to of planting and maintaining container gardens and aesthetic arranging
"Grow All You Can Eat in Three Square Feet"	Editor: Kate Johnsen	innovative solutions to space constraints

"Container Gardening for All Seasons"	Barbara Wise	unique plant suggestions and design ideas across seasons
"The Water-Saving Garden"	Pam Penick	environmentally sustainable practices
"Small-Space Container Gardens"	Fern Richardson	transforming small spaces into vibrant, lush areas
"The Container Gardener's Handbook"	Pippa Greenwood	go-to resource for quick troubleshooting

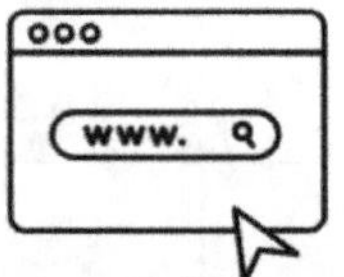

Apps and Websites

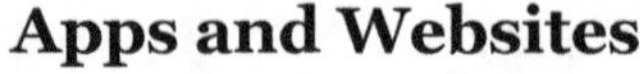

App or Website	Details
PlantNet	allows users to snap a photo of a plant and instantly receive information about its species, care requirements, and more
Waterbot and Garden Manager	reminder of watering schedules, helping to keep plants hydrated without the guesswork
Plantix	diagnosing plant diseases and pests by uploading images of affected plant areas, helps stop disease spread
Gardeners' World and The Spruce	comprehensive articles that cover everything from basic gardening techniques to advanced tips for specific plants, ideal for self-education
GardenWeb and Houzz	platform for community interaction to pose questions, share experiences, and receive advice from fellow gardeners worldwide

Missouri Botanical Garden's Plant Finder	online plant database www.missouribotanicalgarden.org/PlantFinder
USDA's PLANTS Database	online plant database www.plants.usda.gov
Garden Planner and My Garden	digitally visualize and plan garden space, experiment with different plant arrangements, container styles, and garden themes

Local Resources and Communities for Gardeners

Type	Benefits
Gardening Clubs	invaluable networking and resource-sharing avenues, provide nexus for like-minded individuals, collaborative environment, collective purchasing power, supportive with challenges

Nurseries and Garden Centers	treasure troves of quality plants and expert gardening advice, well-educated and enthusiastic staff, advice personalized to local climate and urban garden challenges, locally sourced plants, alerts on new arrivals
Community Gardens	provide opportunities for more physical space through communal spaces, foster a sense of community and collective responsibility, cultivate wider variety of plants, learn from diverse fellow gardeners, promote neighborhood green spaces
Workshops and Classes	further enhance knowledge and skills, workshops from local botanical gardens, nurseries or community colleges, learn sustainability practice and design trends, hands-on classes and feedback from experts, insight into innovations like vertical and hydroponic gardening

Your feedback is greatly appreciated!

Your feedback, support, and reviews make it possible for us to create high-quality books and serve more people.

It only takes 60 seconds to leave an honest review. Share your feedback and thoughts so others can see the quality of this book.

Find the location where you purchased the book and leave a review. Select a rating and write a couple of sentences.

That's it! Thank you so much for your support.

Review this product

Share your thoughts with other customers

References

9 DIY Garden Markers Everyone Should Make! (n.d.). Retrieved July 23, 2025, from https://gharpedia.com/blog/diy-garden-markers-everyone-should-make/

15 Best Zen Garden Ideas on a Budget—Hello Lidy. (n.d.). Pinterest. Retrieved July 23, 2025, from https://www.pinterest.com/pin/465137467781498964/

Amazon.com: 3Pcs 31.5 x 12.6 Inch Peony Cages and Supports, Grow Through Plant Supports for Outdoor Plants, 7mm Metal Peony Support Stakes with Grid Cage, Garden Flower Support Rings Hoops for Large Peonies: Patio, Lawn & Garden. (n.d.). Retrieved July 23, 2025, from https://www.amazon.com/Supports-Through-Outdoor-Support-Peonies/dp/B0DRVR1VN2/ref=sxin_15_pa_sp_search_thematic_sspa?content-id=amzn1.sym.2da95b6c-f59a-4699-bc43-d0ff036c6388%3Aamzn1.sym.2da95b6c-f59a-4699-bc43-d0ff036c6388&crid=1VSRXFVA9S2J3&cv_ct_cx=garden+support+stakes+grow+through&keywords=garden+support+stakes+grow+through&pd_rd_i=B0DRVR1VN2&pd_rd_r=5e3a2fe4-8ab2-43fc-92f6-f17caac0bc26&pd_rd_w=AunUV&pd_rd_wg=OoYxb&pf_rd_p=2da95b6c-f59a-4699-bc43-d0ff036c6388&pf_rd_r=X8SHJB1FJPV2SD5AM4P3&qid=1753311799&sbo=RZvfv%2F%2FHxDF%2BO5021pAnSA%3D%3D&sprefix=garden+support+stakes+grow+throug%2Caps%2C207&sr=1-2-6024b2a3-78e4-4fed-8fed-e1613be3bcce-

spons&sp_csd=d2lkZ2V0TmFtZT1zcF9zZWFyY2hfdGhlb WF0aWM&psc=1

Amazon.com: Balcony Buddies Railing Planter for Outdoor Plants (6-inch, 3-Pack) | Hanging Planter for Railings, Fence Posts | Balcony Wall Planter for Herbs, Flowers and Succulents | Made in The USA : Patio, Lawn & Garden. (n.d.). Retrieved July 23, 2025, from https://www.amazon.com/Balcony-Buddies-Railing-Planter-Outdoor/dp/B09XN9G9GC/ref=sr_1_1_sspa?dib=eyJ2Ij oiMSJ9.Ktj_hcQOjtxA4nYP5ifftgLVkdGDlfXy081xNwwB dvLrixvU48kvV_MDXUPEGefESSXnoZynsfQBvtKcuc5k8 rj_W84SOTdw8m9q23mizOfRsI1AQDr7hCsX8vVBWo6 WMwpB3qRiOpBVfG9zqFVHNLgi9bZ-sPtgRX0LxJ6Ce4b8wd19WeurCkagE6vSAMQgqtt5fBgnl1 BjVzEkIKt0IolvXC-4qluaSCsThYlyDB3G1pvZltBQWsLf2S2ye1zb6A6mdv-YpKjs-YRWLQ_wEPiTdMv-t6ZyLv6p8fc5ap8.kwzCCQx8ItgjKRKG-00qlPdA51ovrKEmPTy2HwSo0Qk&dib_tag=se&keyword s=balcony%2Bbuddies%2Brailing%2Bplanter%2Boutdoor &qid=1753310290&sr=8-1-spons&sp_csd=d2lkZ2V0TmFtZT1zcF9hdGY&th=1

Amazon.com: Breeze Touch 2 Pack Tomato Support Cages, Up to 59 Inch Adjustable Tomato Trellis for Garden & Pots, Garden Trellis for Climbing Plants Outdoor, Plant Trellis for Climbing Vegetables, Flowers, Beans: Patio, Lawn & Garden. (n.d.). Retrieved July 23, 2025, from https://www.amazon.com/Breeze-Touch-Adjustable-Climbing-Vegetables/dp/B0DPLXRHZT/ref=sr_1_25?dib=eyJ2Ijoi MSJ9.PAlo9IDHdVI1s3PYns7YtsNv9G4l95E_XrE0YG8T mWSM-uXWqtg-

LqjMyjOdduy0BdYcCeqh79MwWcekThQX9aoK9j62nnsO
q4ku-
hmMejgOapGFtvxr82YSzDvDGM7iu2swb3FCltvUApVfB
QLTamp3hf0B_a8A5gGW7ITs-
TOflkdnjhw6zY2OhOSAHr8KPGuL9AIuiELRZaEKGuM7
Fs2ZLE0-OeUohm1iPRj1ei9hAl8RM2PsaWaAi-jb6vHcw-
J3vd0VA6-
OZoJnWui7XZpg14iZdXDBYYxbUwFlaAw.EKWDECUDf
FmOiihlT7C93EPnA41DEMl5dofphnuFyGI&dib_tag=se&
keywords=trellis%2Bsupports%2Bclimbing%2Boutdoor%
2Bvegetable&qid=1753311631&sr=8-25&th=1

*Amazon.com: Plant Stake Support—6 Pack, Garden Single Stem
Support Stake Plant Cage Support Rings, Single Stem
Plant Support Stakes, Plant Twist Ties, for Flowers
Amaryllis Tomatoes Peony Lily Rose (15.9 inch): Patio,
Lawn & Garden.* (n.d.). Retrieved July 23, 2025,
from https://www.amazon.com/Plant-Stake-Support-
Amaryllis-
Tomatoes/dp/B08395DRVF/ref=sr_1_7?dib=eyJ2IjoiMS
J9.dOBtx1xmBkej94qHMtzeBmUwPTf_9UHRdamAqZs7
021tSbJJh2eHhbv_x6E-
wbhZzBJLcZkVcF9Brg0txGapfGqGyERRiX1zbKsi2GyAPP
t1nC2G8ce76foRkg1Yhkeya6QOXRvRnOoei62LHXtY4Tn
PG0oPbAMKz_WsptIcOV9rkkAOLLaEP-
CjNWHrXJwtiGvetm5duU1gqL8wtVJExy_Jpo5QtUJYz0
ZCamMvMrszuI2LJ9NXmIQt2x03ycckHX5k1_oR_A-
ktOK6bbiHeEgB4jbbcb6uJducE4k6JME.IZvGm1V0-
ICeSwR9FnQVShICDrCPctIgRQ_PAowmONM&dib_tag=
se&keywords=stakes%2Bsingle%2Bsupport%2Brosemary
%2Bplants&qid=1753311388&sr=8-7&th=1

Butler, A. (2020, October 15). 12 Vertical Gardening Ideas to Turn
Your Small Space Into an Outdoor Paradise. *Lawnstarter*.

https://www.lawnstarter.com/blog/landscaping/vertical-gardening-ideas/

Childs, J. (2021, July 14). *Prune Spring Flowering Shrubs for More Flowers*. Garden Gate. https://www.gardengatemagazine.com/articles/how-to/prune/prune-spring-flowering-shrubs-for-more-flowers/

Container Gardening for Beginners: 10 Steps for Success—Growing In The Garden. (n.d.). Retrieved July 23, 2025, from https://growinginthegarden.com/container-gardening-for-beginners-10-steps-for-success/

Designer, N. S. | P. (2023, March 21). *Container Garden Companion Planting Guide*. Permaculture Apart. https://www.permacultureapartment.com/post/container-garden-companion-planting

DIY 4-Tower Kit (recirculating). (n.d.). Retrieved July 23, 2025, from https://mrstacky.com/diy-4-tower-kit-recirculating.html

Dr.meter Soil Moisture Meter, S10 Hygrometer Moisture Sensor for Garden, Farm, Lawn Plants Indoor & Outdoor(No Battery needed). (n.d.). Dr.Meter. Retrieved July 23, 2025, from https://drmeter.com/products/s10-soil-moisture-meter

FS055: Container Gardening with Vegetables (Rutgers NJAES). (n.d.). Retrieved July 23, 2025, from https://njaes.rutgers.edu/FS055/

Herbal—Vertical gardens—Urban farming in the microscale | My4ns.com. (n.d.). Retrieved July 23, 2025, from https://4naturesystem.com/en/blog/bid-52-herbal-vertical-gardens-urban-farming-microscale

HGTV.com, D. T. F. D. on: A. a contributor to, woodworking, D. develops design-forward D. projects for anyone looking to advance their skills in, welding, & Improvement, H.

(n.d.). *How to Build a Hoop House to Protect Your Vegetables*. HGTV. Retrieved July 23, 2025, from https://www.hgtv.com/outdoors/gardens/how-to-build-a-hoop-house-to-protect-your-vegetables

How to secure planter baskets to balcony railings? (n.d.). Retrieved July 23, 2025, from https://getpotted.com/inspiration/gardening-tips/how-to-secure-planter-baskets-to-balcony-railings/

Knight, C. (2021, April 27). DIY Solar Water Fountain Under $50, *Southern Chick Journal*. http://www.southernchickjournal.com/2021/04/27/diy-solar-water-fountain-under-50/

Krause, T. (2019). *English: A very useful map for determining world hardiness zones*. [Graphic]. https://www.pinterest.co.uk/pin/361836151281599507/. https://commons.wikimedia.org/w/index.php?curid=83615430

Lisa. (2020, June 9). *My Gardening Journey – How to Thin Seedlings—Simple Eco Mama*. https://simpleecomama.com/my-gardening-journey-how-to-thin-seedlings/, https://simpleecomama.com/my-gardening-journey-how-to-thin-seedlings/

Magazine, B. G. W. (n.d.). *Best Plants for Balconies | BBC Gardeners World Magazine*. Retrieved July 23, 2025, from https://www.gardenersworld.com/plants/best-plants-for-balconies/

Pinching-pruning.jpg (736×358). (n.d.). Retrieved July 23, 2025, from https://www.aldenlane.com/m/wp-content/uploads/2015/07/pinching-pruning.jpg

Pollinator-Friendly Native Plant Lists. (n.d.). Xerces Society. Retrieved July 23, 2025, from https://xerces.org/pollinator-conservation/pollinator-friendly-plant-lists

Project—Automatic drip irrigation for a balcony garden. (n.d.). Retrieved July 23, 2025, from http://topazturtlehandmade.blogspot.com/2016/02/project-automatic-drip-irrigation-for.html

Raised Bed Garden Kit | Rain Bird. (n.d.). Retrieved July 23, 2025, from https://www.rainbird.com/products/raised-bed-garden-kit

Rent.com. (n.d.). *How to Make a Compost Pile in a Small Apartment.* Forbes. Retrieved July 23, 2025, from https://www.forbes.com/sites/rent/2014/04/12/how-to-make-a-compost-pile-in-a-small-apartment/

Sakawsky, A. (2019, March 29). *How to Build a DIY Row Cover to Extend Your Growing Season.* https://thehouseandhomestead.com/diy-row-cover/

Stephy. (2023, June 29). 60 DIY Vertical Garden Ideas for Small Spaces. *Prudent Penny Pincher.* https://www.prudentpennypincher.com/vertical-garden-ideas-for-small-spaces/

Urban Farming with Drip Irrigation. (n.d.). DripWorks. Retrieved July 23, 2025, from https://www.dripworks.com/blog/urban-farming-with-drip-irrigation

Urban Gardening: Growing Plants & Vegetation in the City. (n.d.). Retrieved July 23, 2025, from https://www.ambius.com/resources/blog/plant-care/urban-gardening-tips

USDA Plant Hardiness Zone Map. (n.d.). Retrieved July 23, 2025, from https://planthardiness.ars.usda.gov/

W, E. (2019, August 13). The Benefits of Mulch—More Than Just Decoration! -. *1 Stop Landscape*

Supply. https://1stoplandscapefl.com/the-benefits-of-mulch/

What are the differences in usage between anvil and bypass pruner—Knowledge. (n.d.). Retrieved July 23, 2025, from https://www.rhinogardening.com/info/the-difference-between-anvil-and-bypass-pruner-77010342.html